Teen Health Series

# Tobacco Information For Teens, Third Edition

# Tobacco Information For Teens,
# Third Edition

Health Tips About The Hazards Of
Using Cigarettes, Smokeless Tobacco,
And Other Nicotine Products

Including Facts About Nicotine Addiction, Nicotine
Delivery Systems, Secondhand Smoke, Health Consequences
Of Tobacco Use, Related Cancers, Smoking Cessation,
And Tobacco Use Statistics

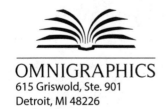

OMNIGRAPHICS
615 Griswold, Ste. 901
Detroit, MI 48226

Bibliographic Note

Because this page cannot legibly accommodate all the copyright notices, the Bibliographic Note portion of the Preface constitutes an extension of the copyright notice.

* * *

Omnigraphics
a part of Relevant Information
Keith Jones, *Managing Editor*

* * *

Library of Congress Cataloging-in-Publication Data

Names: Omnigraphics, Inc.

Title: Tobacco information for teens: health tips about the hazards of using cigarettes, smokeless tobacco, and other nicotine products: including facts about nicotine addiction, nicotine delivery systems, secondhand smoke, health consequences of tobacco use, related cancers, smoking cessation, and tobacco use statistics.

Description: Third edition. | Detroit, MI: Omnigraphics, [2017] | Series: Teen health series | Includes bibliographical references and index. | Audience: Grade 9 to 12.

Identifiers: LCCN 2016054311 (print) | LCCN 2016057261 (ebook) | ISBN 9780780813878 (hardcover: alk. paper) | ISBN 9780780814134 (ebook) | ISBN 9780780814134 (eBook)

Subjects: LCSH: Tobacco use--Health aspects. | Smoking--Health aspects. | Nicotine--Health aspects. | Smoking cessation. | Teenagers--Tobacco use--Prevention.

Classification: LCC RA1242.T6 T615 2017 (print) | LCC RA1242.T6 (ebook) | DDC 613.850835--dc23

LC record available at https://lccn.loc.gov/2016054311

# Table of Contents

# Part Three: Cancers Associated With Tobacco Use

# Part Four: Other Health Concerns Related To Tobacco Use

# Part Five: Tobacco Use Cessation

# Part Six: If You Need More Help Or Information

# Preface

## About This Book

Tobacco use is the leading cause of preventable disease and death in the United States. According to a recent report from the U.S. Department of Health and Human Services nearly 90 percent of adult smokers began smoking before the age of 18. And while tobacco use by adolescents has declined substantially in the last 40 years, nearly 4.7 million middle and high school students were tobacco users in 2015. The health consequences of tobacco use can be devastating. Cigarette smoking by young people can lead to immediate and serious health problems, including respiratory and cardiovascular effects, changes in brain chemistry, and risks for nicotine addiction. Long-term smoking is linked to a host of life threatening disorders, including various cancers, lung diseases, and heart attacks. In fact, according to statistics from the Centers for Disease Control and Prevention (CDC), cigarettes cause more than 480,000 premature deaths in the United States each year—from smoking or exposure to secondhand smoke—about 1 in every 5 U.S. deaths.

*Tobacco Information For Teens*, Third Edition, offers updated information about the health consequences associated with smoking and other forms of tobacco use. It explains some of the cultural influences that can make tobacco use seem attractive and how teen curiosity can lead to nicotine-related problems. The various methods by which nicotine is consumed, including different types of cigarettes, cigars, hookah pipes, smokeless products, and even secondhand smoke, are explained. A section on cancers associated with tobacco describes the organs most commonly affected. A section on other health concerns related to tobacco use discusses some of the most common smoking-related diseases, including those that impact the heart, lungs, circulatory system, eyes, and sex organs. For teens who want to stop smoking—or help a friend or family member quit—facts about smoking cessation are included along with tips for dealing with the effects of nicotine withdrawal. The book concludes with directories of resources for more information.

## How To Use This Book

This book is divided into parts and chapters. Parts focus on broad areas of interest; chapters are devoted to single topics within a part.

*Part One: Facts About Tobacco And Nicotine* provides data about the use of tobacco and other nicotine products. It explains how nicotine use leads to addiction, and it offers statistical information about the use of nicotine products in the United States and around the world. It also discusses legislative action concerning the sale and marketing of tobacco products.

*Part Two: Nicotine Delivery Systems* offers facts about the most common ways people consume or are exposed to nicotine. These include smoking different kinds of cigarettes, cigars, and pipes, using smokeless tobacco, and breathing secondhand smoke. Information on more recent nicotine delivery systems such as e-cigarettes and hookah pipes are also discussed.

*Part Three: Cancers Associated With Tobacco Use* provides basic information about the types of cancer for which risks are most commonly linked to tobacco use. Although lung cancer is perhaps the most widely recognized cancer-related risk, others include bladder cancer, esophageal cancer, laryngeal cancer, oral cancer, and pancreatic cancer.

*Part Four: Other Health Concerns Related To Tobacco Use* explains how smoking and other tobacco use can lead to disease processes other than cancer that also harm the body's organs and systems. It discusses tobacco-related damage to the lungs, heart, blood vessels, and eyes, as well as adverse affects on sexual health and pregnancy outcomes.

*Part Five: Tobacco Use Cessation* offers information about quitting smoking or other types of tobacco use. It explains the use of nicotine replacement therapies, discusses medications commonly prescribed to aid in cessation efforts, and offers tips for coping with the effects of nicotine withdrawal.

*Part Six: If You Need More Help Or Information* provides directories of resources for obtaining more information about the health effects of tobacco use and smoking cessation.

## Bibliographic Note

This volume contains documents and excerpts from publications issued by the following U.S. government agencies: Centers for Disease Control and Prevention (CDC); National Cancer Institute (NCI); National Heart, Lung, and Blood Institute (NHLBI); National Institute of Arthritis and Musculoskeletal and Skin Diseases (NIAMS); National Institute of Diabetes and Digestive and Kidney Diseases (NIDDK); National Institute of Dental and Craniofacial Research (NIDCR); National Institute on Drug Abuse (NIDA); U.S. Department of Health and Human Services (HHS); U.S. Environmental Protection Agency (EPA); U.S. Food and Drug Administration (FDA); and U.S. House of Representatives.

The photograph on the front cover is © mixmike/istock.

# Medical Review

Omnigraphics contracts with a team of qualified, senior medical professionals who serve as medical consultants for the *Teen Health Series*. As necessary, medical consultants review reprinted and originally written material for currency and accuracy. Citations including the phrase, Reviewed (month, year)" indicate material reviewed by this team. Medical consultation services are provided to the *Teen Health Series* editors by:

Dr. Senthil Selvan, MBBS, DCH, MD
Dr. K. Sivanandham, MBBS, DCH, MS (Research), PhD

# About The *Teen Health Series*

At the request of librarians serving today's young adults, the *Teen Health Series* was developed as a specially focused set of volumes within Omnigraphics' *Health Reference Series*. Each volume deals comprehensively with a topic selected according to the needs and interests of people in middle school and high school. Teens seeking preventive guidance, information about disease warning signs, medical statistics, and risk factors for health problems will find answers to their questions in the *Teen Health Series*. The *Series*, however, is not intended to serve as a tool for diagnosing illness, in prescribing treatments, or as a substitute for the physician/patient relationship. All people concerned about medical symptoms or the possibility of disease are encouraged to seek professional care from an appropriate health care provider.

If there is a topic you would like to see addressed in a future volume of the *Teen Health Series*, please write to:

Editor
*Teen Health Series*
Omnigraphics
615 Griswold, Ste. 901
Detroit, MI 48226

# A Note About Spelling And Style

*Teen Health Series* editors use *Stedman's Medical Dictionary* as an authority for questions related to the spelling of medical terms and the *Chicago Manual of Style* for questions related to grammatical structures, punctuation, and other editorial concerns. Consistent adherence is not always possible, however, because the individual volumes within the *Series* include many documents from a wide variety of different producers and copyright holders, and the editor's primary goal is to present material from each source as accurately as is possible following the terms specified by each document's producer. This sometimes means that information in different chapters or sections may follow other guidelines and alternate spelling authorities.

# Part One
## Facts About Tobacco And Nicotine

# Chapter 1
# Smoking Stinks

The health effects of cigarette smoking have been the subject of intensive investigation since the 1950s. Cigarette smoking is still considered the chief preventable cause of premature disease and death in the United States.

Considerable evidence indicates that the health problems associated with smoking are a function of the duration (years) and the intensity (amount) of use. The younger one begins to smoke, the more likely one is to be a current smoker as an adult. Earlier onset of cigarette smoking and smokeless tobacco use provides more life-years to use tobacco and thereby increases the potential duration of use and the risk of a range of more serious health consequences.

> ## Numbers to Know
> **88 percent:** the number of adult daily smokers smoked their first cigarette before turning 18.
>
> **18 percent:** the (approximate) number of high school students who smoking cigarettes.
>
> *(Source: "Don't Start Using Tobacco," BeTobaccoFree.gov, November 15, 2012.)*

Earlier onset is also associated with heavier use; those who begin to use tobacco as younger adolescents are among the heaviest users in adolescence and adulthood. Heavier users are more likely to experience tobacco-related health problems and are the least likely to quit smoking cigarettes or using smokeless tobacco. Preventing tobacco use among young people is therefore likely to affect both duration and intensity of total use of tobacco, potentially reducing long-term health consequences significantly.

---

About This Chapter: This chapter includes text excerpted from "Smoking And Tobacco Use," Centers for Disease Control and Prevention (CDC), July 16, 2015.

# Health Consequences Of Tobacco Use Among Young People

Active smoking by young people is associated with significant health problems during childhood and adolescence and with increased risk factors for health problems in adulthood. Cigarette smoking during adolescence appears to reduce the rate of lung growth and the level of maximum lung function that can be achieved. Young smokers are likely to be less physically fit than young nonsmokers; fitness levels are inversely related to the duration and the intensity of smoking. Adolescent smokers report that they are significantly more likely than their nonsmoking peers to experience shortness of breath, coughing spells, phlegm production, wheezing, and overall diminished physical health. Cigarette smoking during childhood and adolescence poses a clear risk for respiratory symptoms and problems during adolescence; these health problems are risk factors for other chronic conditions in adulthood, including chronic obstructive pulmonary disease.

Cardiovascular disease is the leading cause of death among adults in the United States. Atherosclerosis, however, may begin in childhood and become clinically significant by young adulthood. Cigarette smoking has been shown to be a primary risk factor for coronary heart disease, arteriosclerotic peripheral vascular disease, and stroke. Smoking by children and adolescents is associated with an increased risk of early atherosclerotic lesions and increased risk factors for cardiovascular diseases. These risk factors include increased levels of low-density lipoprotein cholesterol, increased very-low-density lipoprotein cholesterol, increased triglycerides, and reduced levels of high-density lipoprotein cholesterol. If sustained into adulthood, these patterns significantly increase the risk for early development of cardiovascular disease.

> Every day, more than 1,200 people in this country die due to smoking. For each of those deaths, at least two youth or young adults become regular smokers each day. Almost 90 percent of those replacement smokers smoke their first cigarette by age 18.
>
> *(Source: "Preventing Tobacco Use Among Youth And Young Adults," Surgeongeneral.gov, March 8, 2012.)*

Smokeless tobacco use is associated with health consequences that range from halitosis to severe health problems such as various forms of oral cancer. Use of smokeless tobacco by young people is associated with early indicators of adult health consequences, including periodontal degeneration, soft tissue lesions, and general systemic alterations. Previous reports have documented that smokeless tobacco use is as addictive for young people as it is for adults.

Another concern is that smokeless tobacco users are more likely than nonusers to become cigarette smokers.

> Prevention efforts must focus on young adults ages 18 through 25, too. Almost no one starts smoking after age 25. Nearly 9 out of 10 smokers started smoking by age 18, and 99 percent started by age 26. Progression from occasional to daily smoking almost always occurs by age 26.
>
> *(Source: "Preventing Tobacco Use Among Youth And Young Adults," Surgeongeneral.gov, March 8, 2012.)*

Among addictive behaviors such as the use of alcohol and other drugs, cigarette smoking is most likely to become established during adolescence. Young people who begin to smoke at an earlier age are more likely than later starters to develop long-term nicotine addiction. Most young people who smoke regularly are already addicted to nicotine, and they experience this addiction in a manner and severity similar to what adult smokers experience. Most adolescent smokers report that they would like to quit smoking and that they have made numerous, usually unsuccessful attempts to quit. Many adolescents say that they intend to quit in the future and yet prove unable to do so.

Those who try to quit smoking report withdrawal symptoms similar to those reported by adults. Adolescents are difficult to recruit for formal cessation programs, and when enrolled, are difficult to retain in the programs. Success rates in adolescent cessation programs tend to be quite low, both in absolute terms and relative to control conditions.

> - Male adolescents are substantially more likely than females to use smokeless tobacco products; about 20 percent of high school males report current use, whereas only about 1 percent of females do. White adolescents are more likely to smoke and to use smokeless tobacco than are black and Hispanic adolescents.
> - Young people from families with lower socioeconomic status, including those adolescents living in single-parent homes, are at increased risk of initiating smoking. Among environmental factors, peer influence seems to be particularly potent in the early stages of tobacco use; the first tries of cigarettes and smokeless tobacco occur most often with peers, and the peer group may subsequently provide expectations, reinforcement, and cues for experimentation.

Tobacco use is associated with a range of problem behaviors during adolescence. Smokeless tobacco or cigarettes are generally the first drug used by young people in a sequence that can include tobacco, alcohol, marijuana, and hard drugs. This pattern does not imply that tobacco use causes other drug use, but rather that other drug use rarely occurs before the use of tobacco. Still, there are a number of biological, behavioral, and social mechanisms by which the use of one drug may facilitate the use of other drugs, and adolescent tobacco users are substantially more likely to use alcohol and illegal drugs than are nonusers. Cigarette smokers are also more likely to get into fights, carry weapons, attempt suicide, and engage in high-risk sexual behaviors. These problem behaviors can be considered a syndrome, since involvement in one behavior increases the risk for involvement in others. Delaying or preventing the use of tobacco may have implications for delaying or preventing these other behaviors as well.

# Chapter 2
# What You Need To Know About Smoking

## Debunking The Myths About Tobacco

### Myth 1: Smoking Is Just A Choice

- The first time? Yes. After just a few cigarettes? No.

- Addiction to nicotine can happen quickly. It changes the chemical balance in your brain. Smoking may seem like it's just a choice or a habit. In fact, most people who use tobacco are addicted.

- Breaking nicotine addiction is harder for some people than others. Quitting can take several tries. But don't give up.

- If you need help to quit, ask your doctor about nicotine replacement, medicines, or coaching.

### Myth 2: Filters Make Cigarettes Safer

- Filters do not protect you. They are designed to make smoke particles smaller. That makes nicotine easier to absorb. This increases addiction.

- Cigarettes have been engineered to speed up nicotine's path to your brain. Their design feeds addiction.

About This Chapter: Text beginning with the heading "Debunking The Myths About Tobacco" is excerpted from "Tobacco: Is What You Know About Smoking Wrong?" Centers for Disease Control and Prevention (CDC), 2010. Reviewed December 2016; Text under the heading "The Health Consequences Of Smoking—50 Years Of Progress" is excerpted from "The Health Consequences Of Smoking—50 Years Of Progress," Surgeongeneral. gov, U.S. Department of Health and Human Services (HHS), January 16, 2014.

- Light or low-tar cigarettes may sound less dangerous. They aren't. These misleading labels are no longer allowed.

- No cigarette is safe. Tobacco smoke contains more than 7,000 chemicals. At least 250 are toxic.

## Myth 3: An Occasional Cigarette Is No Big Deal

- Smoking doesn't just cause diseases for heavy smokers or longtime smokers.

- Tobacco smoke can trigger sudden heart attacks and death, even in nonsmokers.

- Each cigarette you smoke hurts your lungs, your blood vessels, and cells throughout your body.

- Smoking a few cigarettes a week can cause a heart attack.

- Cutting back is not enough to protect you. You have to quit entirely.

## Myth 4: It's Too Late To Quit—The Damage Is Already Done

- It's true that the longer you use tobacco, the more you hurt your body. But at any age, the sooner you quit, the sooner your health can improve.

- Within 20 minutes after quitting, your body starts to heal.

- After 2 to 5 years, your risk for stroke is similar to that of a nonsmoker.

- In 10 years, your lung cancer risk is cut in half.

## Myth 5: Secondhand Smoke May Bother People, But It Isn't Dangerous

- Tens of thousands of nonsmokers die every year from breathing others' secondhand smoke.

- Breathing the chemicals in tobacco smoke changes your blood's chemistry almost immediately. Deadly clots can form and block arteries to your heart or brain.

- When you smoke at work, home, or at a restaurant, everyone there breathes poisons.

- If you smoke in your car, rolling down a window does not protect your passengers.

- It is not healthy to breathe any amount of tobacco smoke.

## Myth 6: The Little Bit Of Smoke That Kids Get Doesn't Hurt Them

- Children can get bronchitis, pneumonia, and ear infections from smoke.

- Even if smoking is done by an open window, some of the smoke stays in your house and poisons the air children breathe.

- Children with asthma can have a serious, even deadly, asthma attack from breathing secondhand smoke.

- If you or someone else in your household are not ready to quit, be sure to make your home and car 100 percent smokefree.

# The Health Consequences Of Smoking—50 Years Of Progress

- The century-long epidemic of cigarette smoking has caused an enormous avoidable public health tragedy. Since the first Surgeon General's report in 1964 more than 20 million premature deaths can be attributed to cigarette smoking.

- The tobacco epidemic was initiated and has been sustained by the aggressive strategies of the tobacco industry, which has deliberately misled the public on the risks of smoking cigarettes.

- Since the 1964 Surgeon General's report, cigarette smoking has been causally linked to diseases of nearly all organs of the body, to diminished health status, and to harm to the fetus. Even 50 years after the first Surgeon General's report, research continues to newly identify diseases caused by smoking, including such common diseases as diabetes mellitus, rheumatoid arthritis, and colorectal cancer.

- Exposure to secondhand tobacco smoke has been causally linked to cancer, respiratory, and cardiovascular diseases, and to adverse effects on the health of infants and children.

- . The disease risks from smoking by women have risen sharply over the last 50 years and are now equal to those for men for lung cancer, chronic obstructive pulmonary disease, and cardiovascular diseases.

- In addition to causing multiple diseases, cigarette smoking has many other adverse effects on the body, such as causing inflammation and impairing immune function.

- Although cigarette smoking has declined significantly since 1964, very large disparities in tobacco use remain across groups defined by race, ethnicity, educational level, and socioeconomic status and across regions of the country.

- Since the 1964 Surgeon General's report, comprehensive tobacco control programs and policies have been proven effective for controlling tobacco use. Further gains can be made with the full, forceful, and sustained use of these measures.

- The burden of death and disease from tobacco use in the United States is overwhelmingly caused by cigarettes and other combusted tobacco products; rapid elimination of their use will dramatically reduce this burden.

# Chapter 3
# Chemicals In Tobacco Smoke

The Food, Drug and Cosmetic Act (FD&C Act) requires tobacco manufacturers and importers to report the levels of harmful and potentially harmful constituents (HPHCs) found in their tobacco products and tobacco smoke. HPHCs are chemicals or chemical compounds in tobacco products or tobacco smoke that cause or could cause harm to smokers or nonsmokers.

The U.S. Food and Drug Administration (FDA) must publish HPHC quantities in each brand and subbrand of tobacco product, in a way that people find understandable and not misleading. There are several efforts under way at FDA to make progress toward that goal.

## Preliminary HPHC List

FDA has established a list of harmful and potentially harmful constituents (HPHCs) in tobacco products and tobacco smoke (the established HPHC list) as required by the FD&C Act.

The established list of 93 HPHCs is included in the notice and in the table below.

About This Chapter: Text in this chapter begins with excerpts from "Harmful And Potentially Harmful Constituents (HPHCs)," U.S. Food and Drug Administration (FDA), November 8, 2016; Text under the heading "Communicating To The Public" is excerpted from "Issue Snapshot: Harmful And Potentially Harmful Constituents (HPHCs) In Tobacco Products," U.S. Food and Drug Administration (FDA), January 2015.

**Table 3.1.** Established List Of The Chemicals And Chemical Compounds Identified By FDA As Harmful And Potentially Harmful Constituents In Tobacco Products And Tobacco Smoke

| Constituent | Carcinogen (CA), Respiratory Toxicant (RT), Cardiovascular Toxicant (CT), Reproductive or Developmental Toxicant (RDT), Addictive (AD) |
|---|---|
| Acetaldehyde | CA, RT, AD |
| Acetamide | CA |
| Acetone | RT |
| Acrolein | RT, CT |
| Acrylamide | CA |
| Acrylonitrile | CA, RT |
| Aflatoxin B1 | CA |
| 4-Aminobiphenyl | CA |
| 1-Aminonaphthalene | CA |
| 2-Aminonaphthalene | CA |
| Ammonia | RT |
| Anabasine | AD |
| o-Anisidine | CA |
| Arsenic | CA, CT, RDT |
| A-α-C (2-Amino-9H-pyrido[2,3-b]indole) | CA |
| Benz[a]anthracene | CA, CT |
| Benz[j]aceanthrylene | CA |
| Benzene | CA, CT, RDT |
| Benzo[b]fluoranthene | CA, CT |
| Benzo[k]fluoranthene | CA, CT |
| Benzo[b]furan | CA |
| Benzo[a]pyrene | CA |
| Benzo[c]phenanthrene | CA |
| Beryllium | CA |
| 1,3-Butadiene | CA, RT, RDT |
| Cadmium | CA, RT, RDT |
| Caffeic acid | CA |
| Carbon monoxide | RDT |

**Table 3.1.** Continued

| Constituent | Carcinogen (CA), Respiratory Toxicant (RT), Cardiovascular Toxicant (CT), Reproductive or Developmental Toxicant (RDT), Addictive (AD) |
|---|---|
| Catechol | CA |
| Chlorinated dioxins/furans | CA, RDT |
| Chromium | CA, RT, RDT |
| Chrysene | CA, CT |
| Cobalt | CA, CT |
| Coumarin | Banned in food |
| Cresols (o-, m-, and p-cresol) | CA, RT |
| Crotonaldehyde | CA |
| Cyclopenta[c,d]pyrene | CA |
| Dibenz[a,h]anthracene | CA |
| Dibenzo[a,e]pyrene | CA |
| Dibenzo[a,h]pyrene | CA |
| Dibenzo[a,i]pyrene | CA |
| Dibenzo[a,l]pyrene | CA |
| 2,6-Dimethylaniline | CA |
| Ethyl carbamate (urethane) | CA, RDT |
| Ethylbenzene | CA |
| Ethylene oxide | CA, RT, RDT |
| Formaldehyde | CA, RT |
| Furan | CA |
| Glu-P-1 (2-Amino-6-methyldipyrido[1,2-a:3′,2′-d]imidazole) | CA |
| Glu-P-2 (2-Aminodipyrido[1,2-a:3′,2′-d]imidazole) | CA |
| Hydrazine | CA, RT |
| Hydrogen cyanide | RT, CT |
| Indeno[1,2,3-cd]pyrene | CA |
| IQ (2-Amino-3-methylimidazo[4,5-f]quinoline) | CA |
| Isoprene | CA |
| Lead | CA, CT, RDT |

**Table 3.1.** Continued

| Constituent | Carcinogen (CA), Respiratory Toxicant (RT), Cardiovascular Toxicant (CT), Reproductive or Developmental Toxicant (RDT), Addictive (AD) |
| --- | --- |
| MeA-α-C (2-Amino-3-methyl)-9H-pyrido[2,3-b]indole) | CA |
| Mercury | CA, RDT |
| Methyl ethyl ketone | RT |
| 5-Methylchrysene | CA |
| 4-(Methylnitrosamino)-1-(3-pyridyl)-1-butanone (NNK) | CA |
| Naphthalene | CA, RT |
| Nickel | CA, RT |
| Nicotine | RDT, AD |
| Nitrobenzene | CA, RT, RDT |
| Nitromethane | CA |
| 2-Nitropropane | CA |
| N-Nitrosodiethanolamine (NDELA) | CA |
| N-Nitrosodiethylamine | CA |
| N-Nitrosodimethylamine (NDMA) | CA |
| N-Nitrosomethylethylamine | CA |
| N-Nitrosomorpholine (NMOR) | CA |
| N-Nitrosonornicotine (NNN) | CA |
| N-Nitrosopiperidine (NPIP) | CA |
| N-Nitrosopyrrolidine (NPYR) | CA |
| N-Nitrososarcosine (NSAR) | CA |
| Nornicotine | AD |
| Phenol | RT, CT |
| PhIP (2-Amino-1-methyl-6-phenylimidazo[4,5-b]pyridine) | CA |
| Polonium-210 | CA |
| Propionaldehyde | RT, CT |
| Propylene oxide | CA, RT |
| Quinoline | CA |
| Selenium | RT |

**Table 3.1.** Continued

| Constituent | Carcinogen (CA), Respiratory Toxicant (RT), Cardiovascular Toxicant (CT), Reproductive or Developmental Toxicant (RDT), Addictive (AD) |
|---|---|
| Styrene | CA |
| o-Toluidine | CA |
| Toluene | RT, RDT |
| Trp-P-1 (3-Amino-1,4-dimethyl-5H-pyrido[4,3-b]indole) | CA |
| Trp-P-2 (1-Methyl-3-amino-5H-pyrido[4,3-b]indole) | CA |
| Uranium-235 | CA, RT |
| Uranium-238 | CA, RT |
| Vinyl acetate | CA, RT |
| Vinyl chloride | CA |

# Tobacco Industry Reporting Requirements

FDA issued draft guidance in 2012 that identified a subset of 20 HPHCs for which manufacturers and importers are to test and report to FDA. FDA chose these 20 because testing methods were well established and widely available. This includes reporting on HPHC levels in three categories of tobacco products: cigarettes (including smoke and filler), smokeless tobacco (such as snuff, plug, chew, loose leaf, and snus), and roll-your-own tobacco.

# Communicating To The Public

Historically, people have learned about tobacco product constituents from advertising and tobacco product labeling. Some studies indicate that people were misled by information about levels of product constituents and their misunderstanding may have made them less likely to quit smoking. FDA carefully considered this when developing research into how consumers perceive and understand levels of tobacco product constituents.

In August 2013, TPSAC met with FDA's Risk Communication Advisory Committee. This joint committee agreed that the methods for displaying the HPHC information that FDA had available could be difficult to understand or be misleading. The committee recommended to delay making a list of HPHC quantities by brand and subbrand available to the public until FDA had conducted more studies about how well people understand such

HPHC information and how their beliefs affect their behavior. FDA recently partnered with the National Institutes of Health (NIH) to fund research that will support the development of understandable and accurate public information about levels of HPHCs in tobacco products.

FDA continues this important research into how best to communicate HPHC amounts in each brand and subbrand of tobacco product. In the meantime, they continue to include messages about harmful and potentially harmful chemicals from tobacco products or smoke in their ongoing public health campaigns.

# Chapter 4
# Smoking's Immediate Effects On The Body

The effects of smoking are serious. It can harm nearly every organ of the body. It causes nearly one of every five deaths in the United States each year.

## How Does Smoking Affect My Body's Immune System?

The immune system is the body's way of protecting itself from infection and disease. Smoking compromises the immune system, making smokers more likely to have respiratory infections.

Smoking also causes several autoimmune diseases, including Crohn's disease and rheumatoid arthritis. It may also play a role in periodic flare-ups of signs and symptoms of autoimmune diseases. Smoking doubles your risk of developing rheumatoid arthritis.

Smoking has recently been linked to type 2 diabetes, also known as adult-onset diabetes. Smokers are 30 percent to 40 percent more likely to develop type 2 diabetes than nonsmokers. Additionally, the more cigarettes an individual smokes, the higher the risk for diabetes.

## How Does Smoking Affect My Bones?

Recent studies show a direct relationship between tobacco use and decreased bone density. Smoking is one of many factors—including weight, alcohol consumption, and activity

About This Chapter: This chapter includes text excerpted from "Effects Of Smoking On Your Health," BeTobaccoFree.gov, U.S. Department of Health and Human Services (HHS), November 11, 2016.

level—that increase your risk for osteoporosis, a condition in which bones weaken and become more likely to fracture.

Significant bone loss has been found in older women and men who smoke. Quitting smoking appears to reduce the risk for low bone mass and fractures. However, it may take several years to lower a former smoker's risk.

In addition, smoking from an early age puts women at even higher risk for osteoporosis. Smoking lowers the level of the hormone *estrogen* in your body, which can cause you to go through menopause earlier, boosting your risk for osteoporosis.

# How Does Smoking Affect My Heart And Blood Vessels?

The chemicals in tobacco smoke harm your blood cells and damage the function of your heart. This damage increases your risk for:

- Atherosclerosis, a disease in which a waxy substance called plaque builds up in your arteries.

- Aneurysms, which are bulging blood vessels that can burst and cause death.

- Cardiovascular disease (CVD), which includes:

  - Coronary heart disease (CHD), narrow or blocked arteries around the heart

  - Heart attack and damage to your arteries

  - Heart-related chest pain

  - High blood pressure

- Coronary Heart disease, where platelets—components in the blood—stick together along with proteins for form clots which can then get stuck in the plaque in the walls of arteries and cause heart attacks.

- Peripheral arterial disease (PAD), a condition in which plaque builds up in the arteries that carry blood to the head, organs, and limbs.

- Stroke, which is sudden death of brain cells caused by blood clots or bleeding.

Breathing tobacco smoke can even change your blood chemistry and damage your blood vessels. As you inhale smoke, cells that line your body's blood vessels react to its chemicals. Your heart rate and blood pressure go up and your blood vessels thicken and narrow.

# How Does Smoking Affect My Lungs And Breathing?

Every cigarette you smoke damages your breathing and scars your lungs. Smoking causes:

- Chronic obstructive pulmonary disease (COPD), a disease that gets worse over time and causes wheezing, shortness of breath, chest tightness, and other symptoms.

- Emphysema, a condition in which the walls between the air sacs in your lungs lose their ability to stretch and shrink back. Your lung tissue is destroyed, making it difficult or impossible to breathe.

- Chronic bronchitis, which causes swelling of the lining of your bronchial tubes. When this happens, less air flows to and from your lungs.

- Pneumonia

- Asthma

- Tuberculosis

People with asthma can suffer severe attacks when around cigarette smoke.

# How Does Smoking Affect My Vision?

Smoking is as bad for your eyes as it is for the rest of your body. Research has linked smoking to an increased risk of developing age-related macular degeneration, cataract, and optic nerve damage, all of which can lead to blindness.

# Does Smoking Cause Cancer?

Tobacco smoke contains more than 7,000 chemicals. About 70 of them are known to cause cancer. Smoking cigarettes is the number-one risk factor for lung cancer. But, smoking can affect your entire body, and is known to cause cancer in the:

- Bladder

- Bronchus

- Colon

- Esophagus

- Kidney

- Larynx

- Lip

- Liver

- Lungs

- Nasal Cavity

- Nasopharynx

- Oral Cavity

- Pancreas

- Rectum

- Stomach

- Trachea

- Uterine Cervix

In addition, smoking is known to cause leukemia.

## Does Cigars And Pipes Cause Cancer?

Cigar and pipe smoke, like cigarette smoke, contains toxic and cancer-causing chemicals that are harmful to both smokers and non-smokers. Cigar and pipe smoking causes:

- Bladder cancer

- Esophageal cancer

- Laryngeal (voice box) cancer

- Lip cancer

- Lung cancer

- Mouth cancer

- Throat cancer

- Tongue cancer

If you smoke cigars daily, you are at increased risk for developing heart disease and lung diseases such as emphysema.

# Is There Any Safe Cigarette?

There is no such thing as a safe cigarette. People who smoke any kind of cigarette are at an increased risk for smoking-related diseases. Although it is no longer legal to sell light cigarettes, people who smoked light cigarettes in the past are likely to have inhaled the same amount of toxic chemicals as those who smoked regular cigarettes. They remain at high risk of developing smoking-related cancers and other diseases.

# Are Menthol Cigarettes Safe?

All cigarettes are harmful, including menthol cigarettes. Many smokers think menthol cigarettes are less harmful, but there is no evidence that menthol cigarettes are safer than other cigarettes. Like other cigarettes, menthol cigarettes harm nearly every organ in the body and cause many diseases, including cancer, cardiovascular diseases, and respiratory diseases. Menthol cigarettes, like other cigarettes, also negatively impact male and female fertility and are harmful to pregnant women and their unborn babies.

Some research shows that menthol cigarettes may be more addictive than non-menthol cigarettes. More research is needed to understand how addiction differs between menthol and non-menthol cigarette use.

# Chapter 5
# Nicotine Addiction

Nicotine, a component of tobacco, is the primary reason that tobacco is addictive, although cigarette smoke contains many other dangerous chemicals, including tar, carbon monoxide, acetaldehyde, nitrosamines, and more.

An improved overall understanding of addiction and of nicotine as an addictive drug has been instrumental in developing medications and behavioral treatments for tobacco addiction. For example, the nicotine patch and gum, now readily available at drugstores and supermarkets nationwide, have proven effective for smoking cessation when combined with behavioral therapy.

Advanced neuroimaging technologies make it possible for researchers to observe changes in brain function that result from smoking tobacco. Researchers are now also identifying genes that predispose people to tobacco addiction and predict their response to smoking cessation treatments. These findings—and many other recent research accomplishments—present unique opportunities to discover, develop, and disseminate new treatments for tobacco addiction, as well as scientifically based prevention programs to help curtail the public health burden that tobacco use represents.

There are more than 7,000 chemicals found in the smoke of tobacco products. Of these, nicotine, first identified in the early 1800s, is the primary reinforcing component of tobacco.

Cigarette smoking is the most popular method of using tobacco; however, many people also use smokeless tobacco products, such as snuff and chewing tobacco. These smokeless products also contain nicotine, as well as many toxic chemicals.

About This Chapter: This chapter includes text excerpted from "Tobacco/Nicotine," National Institute on Drug Abuse (NIDA), July 2012. Reviewed December 2016.

The cigarette is a very efficient and highly engineered drug delivery system. By inhaling tobacco smoke, the average smoker takes in 1–2 milligrams of nicotine per cigarette. When tobacco is smoked, nicotine rapidly reaches peak levels in the bloodstream and enters the brain. A typical smoker will take 10 puffs on a cigarette over a period of 5 minutes that the cigarette is lit. Thus, a person who smokes about 1½ packs (30 cigarettes) daily gets 300 "hits" of nicotine to the brain each day. In those who typically do not inhale the smoke—such as cigar and pipe smokers and smokeless tobacco users—nicotine is absorbed through the mucosal membranes and reaches peak blood levels and the brain more slowly.

Immediately after exposure to nicotine, there is a "kick" caused in part by the drug's stimulation of the adrenal glands and resulting discharge of epinephrine (adrenaline). The rush of adrenaline stimulates the body and causes an increase in blood pressure, respiration, and heart rate.

# Is Nicotine Addictive?

Yes. Most smokers use tobacco regularly because they are addicted to nicotine. Addiction is characterized by compulsive drug seeking and abuse, even in the face of negative health consequences. It is well documented that most smokers identify tobacco use as harmful and express a desire to reduce or stop using it, and nearly 35 million of them want to quit each year. Unfortunately, more than 85 percent of those who try to quit on their own relapse, most within a week.

Research has shown how nicotine acts on the brain to produce a number of effects. Of primary importance to its addictive nature are findings that nicotine activates reward pathways—the brain circuitry that regulates feelings of pleasure. A key brain chemical involved in mediating the desire to consume drugs is the neurotransmitter dopamine, and research has shown that nicotine increases levels of dopamine in the reward circuits. This reaction is similar to that seen with other drugs of abuse and is thought to underlie the pleasurable sensations experienced by many smokers. For many tobacco users, long-term brain changes induced by continued nicotine exposure result in addiction.

Nicotine's pharmacokinetic properties also enhance its abuse potential. Cigarette smoking produces a rapid distribution of nicotine to the brain, with drug levels peaking within 10 seconds of inhalation. However, the acute effects of nicotine dissipate quickly, as do the associated feelings of reward, which causes the smoker to continue dosing to maintain the drug's pleasurable effects and prevent withdrawal.

Nicotine withdrawal symptoms include irritability, craving, depression, anxiety, cognitive and attention deficits, sleep disturbances, and increased appetite. These symptoms may begin within a few hours after the last cigarette, quickly driving people back to tobacco use. Symptoms peak within the first few days of smoking cessation and usually subside within a few weeks. For some people, however, symptoms may persist for months.

Although withdrawal is related to the pharmacological effects of nicotine, many behavioral factors can also affect the severity of withdrawal symptoms. For some people, the feel, smell, and sight of a cigarette and the ritual of obtaining, handling, lighting, and smoking the cigarette are all associated with the pleasurable effects of smoking and can make withdrawal or craving worse. Nicotine replacement therapies such as gum, patches, and inhalers may help alleviate the pharmacological aspects of withdrawal; however, cravings often persist. Behavioral therapies can help smokers identify environmental triggers of craving so they can employ strategies to prevent or circumvent these symptoms and urges.

# Chapter 6

# Young People And Tobacco: A Statistical Review

If smoking continues at the current rate among youth in this country, 5.6 million of today's Americans younger than 18 will die early from a smoking-related illness. That's about 1 of every 13 Americans aged 17 years or younger alive today.

## Overall Statistical Data

- Tobacco use is started and established primarily during adolescence.

  - Nearly 9 out of 10 cigarette smokers first tried smoking by age 18, and 99 percent first tried smoking by age 26.

  - Each day in the United States, more than 3,200 youth aged 18 years or younger smoke their first cigarette, and an additional 2,100 youth and young adults become daily cigarette smokers.

- Flavorings in tobacco products can make them more appealing to youth.

  - In 2014, 73 percent of high school students and 56 percent of middle school students who used tobacco products in the past 30 days reported using a flavored tobacco product during that time.

About This Chapter: Text in this chapter begins with excerpts from "Youth And Tobacco Use," Centers for Disease Control and Prevention (CDC), April 14, 2016; Text under the heading "Tobacco Use Among Students" is excerpted from "Tobacco Use Among Middle And High School Students—United States, 2011–2015," Centers for Disease Control and Prevention (CDC), April 14, 2016.

# Factors Associated With Youth Tobacco Use

Factors associated with youth tobacco use include the following:

- Social and physical environments

    - The way mass media show tobacco use as a normal activity can promote smoking among young people.

    - Youth are more likely to use tobacco if they see that tobacco use is acceptable or normal among their peers.

    - High school athletes are more likely to use smokeless tobacco than their peers who are non-athletes.

    - Parental smoking may promote smoking among young people.

- Biological and genetic factors

    - There is evidence that youth may be sensitive to nicotine and that teens can feel dependent on nicotine sooner than adults.

    - Genetic factors may make quitting smoking more difficult for young people.

    - A mother's smoking during pregnancy may increase the likelihood that her offspring will become regular smokers.

- Mental health: There is a strong relationship between youth smoking and depression, anxiety, and stress.

- Personal perceptions: Expectations of positive outcomes from smoking, such as coping with stress and controlling weight, are related to youth tobacco use.

- Other influences that affect youth tobacco use include:

    - Lower socioeconomic status, including lower income or education

    - Lack of skills to resist influences to tobacco use

    - Lack of support or involvement from parents

    - Accessibility, availability, and price of tobacco products

    - Low levels of academic achievement

    - Low self-image or self-esteem

    - Exposure to tobacco advertising

# Reducing Youth Tobacco Use

National, state, and local program activities have been shown to reduce and prevent youth tobacco use when implemented together. They include the following:

- Higher costs for tobacco products (for example, through increased taxes).

- Prohibiting smoking in indoor areas of worksites and public places.

- Raising the minimum age of sale for tobacco products to 21 years, which has recently emerged as a potential strategy for reducing youth tobacco use.

- TV and radio commercials, posters, and other media messages targeted toward youth to counter tobacco product advertisements.

- Community programs and school and college policies and interventions that encourage tobacco-free environments and lifestyles.

- Community programs that reduce tobacco advertising, promotions, and availability of tobacco products.

Some social and environmental factors have been found to be related to lower smoking levels among youth. Among these are:

- Religious participation

- Racial/ethnic pride and strong racial identity

- Higher academic achievement and aspirations

Continued efforts are needed to prevent and reduce the use of all forms of tobacco use among youth.

# Tobacco Use Among Students

Tobacco use is the leading cause of preventable disease and death in the United States; if current smoking rates continue, 5.6 million Americans aged <18 years who are alive today are projected to die prematurely from smoking-related disease. Tobacco use and addiction mostly begin during youth and young adulthood. Centers for Disease Control and Prevention (CDC) and the U.S. Food and Drug Administration (FDA) analyzed data from the 2011–2015 National Youth Tobacco Surveys (NYTS) to determine the prevalence and trends of current use of seven tobacco product types (cigarettes, cigars, smokeless tobacco, electronic cigarettes [e-cigarettes], hookahs [water pipes used to smoke tobacco], pipe tobacco, and bidis [small imported cigarettes wrapped in a tendu leaf]) among U.S. middle (grades 6–8) and high (grades 9–12) school students. In 2015, e-cigarettes were the most commonly used tobacco product among middle (5.3%) and high (16%) school students. During 2011–2015, significant increases in current use of e-cigarettes and hookahs occurred among middle and high school students, whereas current use of conventional tobacco products, such as cigarettes and cigars decreased, resulting in no change in overall tobacco product use. During 2014–2015, current use of e-cigarettes increased among middle school students, whereas current use of hookahs decreased among high school students; in contrast, no change was observed in use of hookahs among middle school students, use of e-cigarettes among high school students, or use of cigarettes, cigars, smokeless tobacco, pipe tobacco, or bidis among middle and high school students. In 2015, an estimated 4.7 million middle and high school students were current tobacco product users, and, therefore, continue to be exposed to harmful tobacco product constituents, including nicotine. Nicotine exposure during adolescence, a critical period for brain development, can cause addiction, might harm brain development, and could lead to sustained tobacco product use among youths. Comprehensive and sustained strategies are warranted to prevent and reduce the use of all tobacco products among U.S. youths.

The NYTS is a cross-sectional, school-based, self-administered, pencil-and-paper questionnaire administered to U.S. middle school and high school students. Information is collected on tobacco control outcome indicators to monitor the impact of comprehensive tobacco control policies and strategies and to inform the FDA's regulatory actions. A three-stage cluster sampling procedure was used to generate a nationally representative sample of U.S. students attending public and private schools in grades 6–12. This report uses data from 5 years of NYTS (2011–2015). Sample sizes and overall response rates for 2011, 2012, 2013, 2014, and 2015 were 18,866 (72.7%), 24,658 (73.6%), 18,406 (67.8%), 22,007 (73.3%), and 17,711 (63.4%), respectively.

> In 2015, one in four high school students and one in 13 middle school students reported current use of any tobacco product (≥1 day in the past 30 days). An estimated 4.7 million high school and middle school students reported current use of any tobacco product.

Participants were asked about current use of cigarettes, cigars, smokeless tobacco, e-cigarettes, hookahs, pipe tobacco, and bidis. Current use for each product was defined as use on ≥1 day during the past 30 days. Current tobacco use was categorized as "any tobacco product use," defined as use of one or more tobacco products in the past 30 days; and "≥2 tobacco product use," defined as use of two or more tobacco products in the past 30 days. Kreteks (sometimes referred to as clove cigarettes) are no longer legally sold in the United States, and were excluded from the definition of current any tobacco product use, consistent with other recent reports. Data were weighted to account for the complex survey design and adjusted for nonresponse; national prevalence estimates with 95 percent confidence intervals and population estimates rounded down to the nearest 10,000 were computed. Estimates for current use in 2015 are presented for any tobacco product use, use of ≥2 tobacco products, and use of each tobacco product, by selected demographics for each school level (high and middle). Results were assessed for the presence of linear and quadratic trends to determine the overall trend present, adjusting for race/ethnicity, sex, and grade; p-value <0.05 was used to determine statistical significance. T-tests were performed to examine differences between estimates from 2014 and 2015; p-values <0.05 were considered statistically significant.

In 2015, 25.3 percent of high school students reported current use of any tobacco product, including 13 percent who reported current use of ≥2 tobacco products. Among all high school students, e-cigarettes (16%) were the most commonly used tobacco product, followed by cigarettes (9.3%), cigars (8.6%), hookahs (7.2%), smokeless tobacco (6%), pipe tobacco (1%), and bidis (0.6%). Males reported higher use of any tobacco, ≥2 tobacco products, e-cigarettes, cigarettes, cigars, smokeless tobacco, and bidis than did females. Among non-Hispanic white and Hispanic high school students, e-cigarettes were the most commonly used tobacco product, whereas among non-Hispanic black high school students, cigars were most commonly used. Cigarette use was higher among non-Hispanic whites than among non-Hispanic blacks; and smokeless tobacco use was higher among non-Hispanic whites than other races.

Among middle school students, current use of any tobacco product and ≥2 tobacco products was 7.4 percent and 3.3 percent, respectively. E-cigarettes (5.3%) were the most commonly used tobacco product by middle school students, followed by cigarettes (2.3%), hookahs (2%), smokeless tobacco (1.8%), cigars (1.6%), pipe tobacco (0.4%), and bidis (0.2%). As was the case among high school students, male middle school students reported higher use of any tobacco product than did females. Hispanic middle school students reported higher use of any tobacco product, use of ≥2 tobacco products, and use of e-cigarettes compared with that of other races/ethnicities.

During 2014–2015, current use of hookahs declined among high school students. Use of all other tobacco products, including e-cigarettes, cigarettes, cigars, and smokeless tobacco remained unchanged during this time period among high school students. Among middle school students, e-cigarette use increased from 3.9 percent in 2014 to 5.3 percent in 2015. Use of other tobacco products, including cigarettes, cigars, hookahs, and smokeless tobacco remained unchanged.

During 2011–2015, among all high school students, significant nonlinear increases were observed for current use of e-cigarettes (1.5% to 16.0%) and hookahs (4.1% to 7.2%). Significant linear decreases were observed for current use of cigarettes (15.8% to 9.3%) and smokeless tobacco (7.9% to 6.0%), and significant nonlinear decreases were observed for current use of cigars (11.6% to 8.6%), pipe tobacco (4% to 1%), and bidis (2.0% to 0.6%). Current use of any tobacco product (24.2% to 25.3%) did not change significantly during 2011–2015. Among middle school students, significant linear increases were observed for current use of e-cigarettes (0.6% to 5.3%) and hookahs (1% to 2%). Significant linear decreases were observed for current use of cigarettes (4.3% to 2.3%), cigars (3.5% to 1.6%), and smokeless tobacco (2.7% to 1.8%), and significant nonlinear decreases were observed for current use of pipe tobacco (2.2% to 0.4%) and bidis (1.7% to 0.2%). There was also a significant nonlinear change in the percentage of middle school students reporting current use of ≥2 tobacco products.

In 2015, an estimated 4.7 million middle and high school students were current users of any tobacco product, over 2.3 million of whom were current users of ≥2 tobacco products. Among middle and high school current tobacco users, 3.0 million used e-cigarettes, 1.6 million used cigarettes, 1.4 million used cigars, 1.2 million used hookahs, and 1.1 million used smokeless tobacco.

# Estimates Of Current Tobacco Use Among Youth

## Cigarettes

- From 2011 to 2015, current cigarette smoking declined among middle and high school students.

  - About 2 of every 100 middle school students (2.3%) reported in 2015 that they smoked cigarettes in the past 30 days—a decrease from 4.3% in 2011.

  - About 9 of every 100 high school students (9.3%) reported in 2015 that they smoked cigarettes in the past 30 days—a decrease from 15.8% in 2011.

## Electronic Cigarettes

- Current use of electronic cigarettes increased among middle and high school students from 2011 to 2015.

  - About 5 of every 100 middle school students (5.3%) reported in 2015 that they used electronic cigarettes in the past 30 days—an increase from 0.6% in 2011.

  - 16 of every 100 high school students (16%) reported in 2015 that they used electronic cigarettes in the past 30 days—an increase from 1.5% in 2011.

## Hookahs

- From 2011 to 2015, current use of hookahs increased among middle and high school students.

  - 2 of every 100 middle school students (2%) reported in 2015 that they had used hookah in the past 30 days—an increase from 1% in 2011.

  - About 7 of every 100 high school students (7.2%) reported in 2015 that they had used hookah in the past 30 days—an increase from 4.1% in 2011.

## Smokeless Tobacco

- In 2015:

  - Nearly 2 of every 100 middle school students (1.8%) reported current use of smokeless tobacco.

  - 6 of every 100 high school students (6%) reported current use of smokeless tobacco.

## All Tobacco Product Use

- In 2015, about 7 of every 100 middle school students (7.4%) and about 25 of every 100 high school students (25.3%) used some type of tobacco product.

- In 2013, nearly 18 of every 100 middle school students (17.7%) and nearly half (46%) of high school students said they had ever tried a tobacco product.

## Use Of Multiple Tobacco Products Is Prevalent Among Youth

- In 2015, about 3 of every 100 middle school students (3.3%) and 13 of every 100 high school students (13%) reported use of two or more tobacco products in the past 30 days.

- In 2013, more than 31 of every 100 high school students (31.4%) said they had ever tried two or more tobacco products.

**Table 6.1.** Tobacco Use* Among High School Students In 2015

| Tobacco Product | Overall | Females | Males |
|---|---|---|---|
| Any tobacco product[†] | 25.30% | 20.30% | 30.00% |
| Electronic cigarettes | 16.00% | 12.80% | 19.00% |
| Cigarettes | 9.30% | 7.70% | 10.70% |
| Cigars | 8.60% | 5.60% | 11.50% |
| Hookahs | 7.20% | 6.90% | 7.40% |
| Smokeless tobacco | 6.00% | 1.80% | 10.00% |
| Pipes | 1.00% | 0.70% | 1.40% |
| Bidis | 0.60% | 0.40% | 0.90% |

*"Use" is determined by respondents indicating that they have used a tobacco product on at least 1 day during the past 30 days.

† "Any tobacco product" includes cigarettes, cigars, smokeless tobacco (including chewing tobacco, snuff, dip, snus, and dissolvable tobacco), tobacco pipes, bidis, hookah, and electronic cigarettes.

**Table 6.2.** Tobacco Use* Among Middle School Students In 2015

| Tobacco Product | Overall | Females | Males |
|---|---|---|---|
| Any tobacco product[†] | 7.40% | 6.40% | 8.30% |
| Electronic cigarettes | 5.30% | 4.80% | 5.90% |
| Cigarettes | 2.30% | 2.20% | 2.30% |
| Hookahs | 2.00% | 2.00% | 1.90% |
| Smokeless tobacco | 1.80% | 1.10% | § |
| Cigars | 1.60% | 1.40% | 1.80% |
| Pipes | 0.40% | - | - |
| Bidis | 0.20% | - | - |

*"Use" is determined by respondents indicating that they have used a tobacco product on at least 1 day during the past 30 days.

† "Any tobacco product" includes cigarettes, cigars, smokeless tobacco (including chewing tobacco, snuff, dip, snus, and dissolvable tobacco), tobacco pipes, bidis, hookah, and electronic cigarettes.

§ Where percentages are missing, sample sizes were less than 50 and thus considered unreliable.

# Chapter 7
# Global Trends In Tobacco Use

Tobacco use is a leading preventable cause of morbidity and mortality, with nearly 6 million deaths caused by tobacco use worldwide every year. Cigarette smoking is the most common form of tobacco use in most countries, and the majority of adult smokers initiate smoking before age 18 years. Limiting access to cigarettes among youths is an effective strategy to curb the tobacco epidemic by preventing smoking initiation and reducing the number of new smokers.

Centers for Disease Control and Prevention (CDC) used the Global Youth Tobacco Survey (GYTS) data from 45 countries to examine the prevalence of current cigarette smoking, purchase of cigarettes from retail outlets, and type of cigarette purchases made among school students aged 13–15 years. The results are presented by the six World Health Organization (WHO) regions: African Region (AFR); Eastern Mediterranean Region (EMR); European Region (EUR); Region of the Americas (AMR); South-East Asian Region (SEAR); and Western Pacific Region (WPR).

Across all 45 countries, the median overall current cigarette smoking prevalence among students aged 13–15 years was 6.8 percent (range = 1.7% [Kazakhstan]–28.9% [Timor-Leste]); the median prevalence among boys was 9.7% (2.0% [Kazakhstan]–53.5% [Timor-Leste]), and among girls was 3.5 percent (0.0% [Bangladesh]–26.3% [Italy]). The proportion of current cigarette smokers aged 13–15 years who reported purchasing cigarettes from a retail outlet

About This Chapter: This chapter includes text excerpted from "Current Cigarette Smoking, Access, And Purchases From Retail Outlets Among Students Aged 13–15 Years—Global Youth Tobacco Survey, 45 Countries, 2013 And 2014," Centers for Disease Control and Prevention (CDC), September 1, 2016.

such as a store, street vendor, or kiosk during the past 30 days ranged from 14.9 percent [Latvia] to 95.1% [Montenegro], and in approximately half the countries, exceeded 50 percent.

## Key Findings

- More than 300 million adults in 70 countries across all WHO regions use smokeless tobacco.
- The largest share, 89 percent, are in South-East Asia. In a few countries, notably India and Bangladesh, smokeless tobacco use is very high and surpasses smoking.
- Among youth and adults, males generally show higher prevalence of use than females.
- The best available estimates indicate that, by volume, 91 percent of ST products sold worldwide are sold through "traditional" markets (cottage industry and custom-made).

*(Source: "2014 Smokeless Tobacco And Public Health: A Global Perspective," National Cancer Institute (NCI), December 18, 2014.)*

In the majority of countries assessed in AFR and SEAR, approximately 40 percent of cigarette smokers aged 13–15 years reported purchasing individual cigarettes. Approximately half of smokers in all but one country assessed in EUR reported purchasing cigarettes in packs. These findings could be used by countries to inform tobacco control strategies in the retail environment to reduce and prevent marketing and sales of tobacco products to youths.

GYTS is a nationally representative school-based, paper-and-pencil, cross-sectional survey of students in school grades associated with ages 13–15 years. GYTS uses a standardized methodology that allows cross-country comparisons. Forty-five countries in which the GYTS is implemented had data available for 2013 or 2014 and were included in this report. Current cigarette smoking was defined as a report by a student that they had smoked cigarettes on at least 1 day in the past 30 days. Among current cigarettes smokers, cigarette purchasing from a retail outlet was defined for the majority of countries as a report of having purchased them from a store or shop, a street vendor, or a kiosk in response to the question: "The last time you smoked cigarettes during the past 30 days, how did you get them?" Past 30-day purchase of cigarettes in packs or as individual sticks was also assessed among current cigarette smokers.

Data were weighted for each country to yield nationally representatives estimates. Country-specific prevalence estimates with corresponding 95 percent confidence intervals were calculated, overall and by sex. Estimates based on sample sizes <35 or relative standard error >30 percent are not shown. A Wilcoxon rank sum test was used to compare the median prevalence estimates between boys and girls in each country. Overall sample sizes ranged from 526 (San

Marino [EUR]) to 9,694 (Bosnia and Herzegovina [EUR]). Response rates ranged from 61.5 percent (Pakistan [EMR]) to 100 percent (Bangladesh [SEAR]).

Cigarette smoking prevalences among youths aged 13–15 years by WHO region ranged from 2.3 percent (Mozambique) to 11.2 percent (Zimbabwe) in AFR, from 3.3 percent (Pakistan) to 11.4 percent (Jordan) in EMR, from 1.7 percent (Kazakhstan) to 23.4 percent (Italy) in EUR, from 3.8 percent (Bahamas) to 7.8 percent (Belize) in AMR, from 2.1 percent (Bangladesh) to 28.9 percent (Timor-Leste) in SEAR, and from 2.5 percent (Vietnam) to 11.0 percent (Northern Mariana Islands) in WPR. Across all countries, the median overall current cigarette smoking prevalence was 6.8 percent (range = 1.7% [Kazakhstan]–28.9% [Timor-Leste]); the median prevalence among boys was 9.7 percent (2.0% [Kazakhstan]–53.5% [Timor-Leste]), and among girls was 3.5 percent (0% [Bangladesh]–26.3% [Italy]).

In 26 of the 45 countries, approximately half of current cigarette smokers aged 13–15 years reported purchasing cigarettes from a retail outlet in the past 30 days; this proportion ranged from 14.9 percent in Latvia to 95.1 percent in Montenegro. The proportion of current cigarette smokers who reported buying cigarettes in packs ranged from 15.2 percent in Bangladesh to 89.8 percent in Serbia, and the proportion of who reported buying cigarettes as individual sticks ranged from 3.6 percent in Greece to 84.8 percent in Bangladesh.

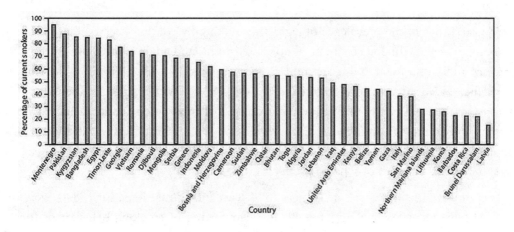

**Figure 7.1.** Global Youth Tobacco Survey

# Discussion

The overall prevalence of cigarette smoking among students aged 13–15 years in the 45 countries included in this report ranged from 1.7 percent (Kazakhstan) to 28.9 percent

(Timor-Leste). Median smoking prevalence was higher among boys than girls. Prevalence also varied among the countries assessed. Reducing youths' access to tobacco products at retail outlets is an effective strategy to reduce smoking by youths. The WHO Framework Convention on Tobacco Control (FCTC) is the first international treaty negotiated under the auspices of WHO, developed in response to the globalization of the tobacco epidemic. Demand reduction measures outlined in FCTC have the potential to protect youths from tobacco use and include tobacco tax increases and bans on tobacco advertising, promotions, and sponsorship. In addition, supply reduction measures such as addressing illicit trade of tobacco products and prohibition of sale of tobacco products to and by minors, also have the potential to reduce the number of youths who smoke.

Forty-three of 45 countries that conducted GYTS in 2013 and 2014 have ratified the FCTC. However, varying levels of tobacco control policy implementation and other country-specific factors can influence cigarette smoking prevalence and access by youths to cigarettes from retail outlets. Challenges in fully implementing Article 16 might include tobacco industry attempts to undermine access laws that aim to reduce use of tobacco among minors, opposition from retailers, poor enforcement, and availability of cigarettes at alternate outlets that are not regulated in some countries. The availability of cigarettes for purchase as single sticks, which was common in some countries, makes purchasing less expensive and more attainable for youths, who are generally sensitive to prices.

The variations in the prevalence of cigarette smoking by youths observed by country and by sex might reflect differences in social norms, customs, and adult tobacco use patterns that influence adolescent tobacco use, and underscore the potential impact of full implementation of evidence-based interventions outlined in the WHO MPOWER package. The MPOWER package outlines policies aimed at reversing the global tobacco epidemic, including implementing and enforcing comprehensive smokefree laws, increasing access to cessation services, warning about the dangers of tobacco use with antismoking media campaigns, and raising taxes to increase the price of tobacco products.

The findings in this report are subject to at least four limitations. First, data were self-reported by students, which might result in misreporting of smoking behavior or tobacco purchasing patterns. Second, students who do not purchase cigarettes themselves might acquire them from other sources such as friends or family. Third, the data presented represent only youths who are enrolled in school, which might limit generalizability to all youths in these countries. Finally, only a limited number of countries were assessed from each WHO region; therefore, the findings in this report do not represent the respective WHO regions overall.

Tobacco prevention and control interventions that restrict youths' access to tobacco products and reduce exposure to youth-oriented tobacco product promotions can reduce tobacco use among youths. Implementing evidence-based measures from FCTC Article 16, in conjunction with evidence-based strategies outlined in WHO's MPOWER package, are critical to reducing the estimated 1 billion tobacco-related deaths projected worldwide this century.

# Chapter 8

# Tobacco Industry Marketing Statistics

## Tobacco Industry Marketing

**Cigarette and smokeless tobacco companies spend billions of dollars each year** to market their products.

- In 2013, cigarette and smokeless tobacco companies spent nearly $9.5 billion on advertising and promotional expenses in the United States alone.

    - Cigarette companies spent approximately $8.95 billion on cigarette advertising and promotion in 2013, down from $9.17 billion in 2012.

    - The five major U.S. smokeless tobacco manufacturers spent $503.2 million on smokeless tobacco advertising and promotion in 2013, an increase from $435.9 million spent in 2012.

**The money cigarette and smokeless tobacco companies spent in 2013 on U.S. marketing amounted to—**

- About $30 million each day

- More than $30 for every person (adults and children) in the United States per year (according to mid-2013 population estimate of 316,000,000)

- More than $228 per year for each U.S. adult smoker (based on 42.1 million adult smokers in 2013)

---

About This Chapter: This chapter includes text excerpted from "Tobacco Industry Marketing," Centers for Disease Control and Prevention (CDC), December 1, 2016.

**The following three categories totaled approximately $8.3 billion and accounted for 93 percent of all cigarette company marketing expenditures in 2013:**

- Price discounts paid to retailers or wholesalers to reduce the price of cigarettes to consumers—$7.6 billion

- Promotional allowances paid to cigarette retailers, such as payments for stocking, shelving, displaying, and merchandising particular brands—$291.3 million

- Promotional allowances paid to cigarette wholesalers, such as payments for volume rebates, incentive payments, value-added services, and promotions—$397.2 million

# Marketing To Specific Populations

## Youth And Young Adults

Scientific evidence shows that tobacco company advertising and promotion influences young people to start using tobacco.

- Adolescents who are exposed to cigarette advertising often find the ads appealing.

- Tobacco ads make smoking appear to be appealing, which can increase adolescents' desire to smoke.

The three most heavily advertised brands—Marlboro, Newport, and Camel—were the preferred brands of cigarettes smoked by adolescents (aged 12–17 years) and young adults (aged 18–25 years) during 2008–2010.

**Brand Preferences of Adolescents:**

- 46.2 percent preferred Marlboro

- 21.8 percent preferred Newport

- 12.4 percent preferred Camel

- 16.0 percent preferred other brands

- 3.5 percent preferred no usual brand

**Brand Preferences of Young Adults:**

- 46.1 percent preferred Marlboro

- 21.8 percent preferred Newport

- 12.4 percent preferred Camel

- 15.2 percent preferred other brands

- 1.6 percent preferred no usual brand

## Women

Women have been targeted by the tobacco industry, and tobacco companies have produced brands specifically for women. Marketing toward women is dominated by themes of social desirability and independence, which are conveyed by advertisements featuring slim, attractive, and athletic models.

## Racial/Ethnic Communities

Advertisement and promotion of certain tobacco products appear to be targeted to members of racial/minority communities.

- Marketing to Hispanics and American Indians/Alaska Natives has included advertising and promotion of cigarette brands with names such as Rio, Dorado, and American Spirit.

- The tobacco industry has targeted African American communities in its advertisements and promotional efforts for menthol cigarettes. Strategies include:

  - Campaigns that use urban culture and language to promote menthol cigarettes

  - Tobacco-sponsored hip-hop bar nights with samples of specialty menthol cigarettes

  - Targeted direct-mail promotions

- Tobacco companies' marketing to Asian Americans has included:

  - Sponsorship of Chinese and Vietnamese New Year festivals and other activities related to Asian/Pacific American Heritage Month

  - Heavy billboard and in-store advertisements in predominantly urban Asian American communities

  - Financial and in-kind contributions to community organizations

  - Support of Asian American business associations

# Chapter 9
# Facts About Tobacco Advertising

## Advertising And Promotion

- Despite the overwhelming evidence of the adverse health effects from tobacco use, efforts to prevent the onset or continuance of tobacco use face the pervasive challenge of promotion activity by the tobacco industry.

- Regulating advertising and promotion, particularly that directed at young people, is very likely to reduce both the prevalence and initiation of smoking.

- The tobacco industry uses a variety of marketing tools and strategies to influence consumer preference, thereby increasing market share and attracting new consumers.

- Among all U.S. manufacturers, the tobacco industry is one of the most intense in marketing its products. Only the automobile industry markets its products more heavily.

## Youth And Tobacco Advertising And Promotion

- Children and teenagers constitute the majority of all new smokers, and the industry's advertising and promotion campaigns often have special appeal to these young people.

- One tobacco company, the Liggett Group, Inc., has admitted that the entire tobacco industry conspired to market cigarettes to children.

About This Chapter: Text beginning with the heading "Advertising And Promotion" is excerpted from "Highlights: Tobacco Advertising And Promotion," Centers for Disease Control and Prevention (CDC), July 21, 2015; Text beginning with the heading "Promotion And Advertising Guidelines" is excerpted from "Advertising And Promotion," U.S. Food and Drug Administration (FDA), November 2, 2016.

- Tobacco documents recently obtained in litigation indicate that tobacco companies have purposefully marketed to children as young as 14 years of age.

- The effect of tobacco advertising on young people is best epitomized by R.J. Reynolds Company's introduction of the Joe Camel campaign. From the introduction of the "Old Joe" cartoon character in 1988, Camel's share of the adolescent cigarette market increased dramatically—from less than 1 percent before 1988, to 8 percent in 1989, to more than 13 percent in 1993.

- In 1997 the Federal Trade Commission (FTC) filed a complaint against R.J. Reynolds alleging that "the purpose of the Joe Camel campaign was to reposition the Camel brand to make it attractive to young smokers" The FTC ultimately dismissed its complaint after the November 23, 1998, Master Settlement Agreement (MSA), which calls for the ban of all cartoon characters, including Joe Camel, in the advertising, promotion, packaging, and labeling of any tobacco product.

---

## Key Findings

- In some high-income countries, tobacco manufacturers have introduced novel smokeless tobacco products, using product innovations such as portion pouches, dissolvable tobacco, unique flavorings, and varying nicotine levels which may make novel products more attractive to consumers, including those who have not previously used smokeless tobacco products. Tobacco manufacturers, including cigarette manufacturers, have marketed new smokeless tobacco products to smokers for use in situations where they cannot smoke or do not want to smoke, such as at work, in smokefree bars, or around family members. These marketing strategies may have an adverse public health impact if they encourage dual use or use of multiple tobacco products, discourage cessation, or encourage new tobacco use initiation.

- In low- and middle-income countries, product innovations may also make sale and use of products more convenient. For example, in India the gutka industry has promoted a packaged ready-to-use product based on a traditional custom-made mixture.

*(Source: "2014 Smokeless Tobacco And Public Health: A Global Perspective," National Cancer Institute (NCI), December 18, 2014.)*

---

# Promotion And Advertising Guidelines

To reduce the number of children and adolescents who use tobacco products and to prevent health consequences associated with tobacco use, the Food, Drug, and Cosmetic Act

(FD & C Act) and its implementing regulations restrict the way tobacco product manufacturers, retailers, and distributors can advertise and promote tobacco products.

---

## When Do Manufacturers Need To Comply?

For newly-regulated tobacco products, the U.S. Food and Drug Administration (FDA) has provided a compliance period for certain labeling and advertising requirements:

- 2016
  - Stop distributing products with modified risk claims (other than "light," "low," or "mild") by August 8, 2016.
- 2017
  - Stop distributing products with modified risk claims, i.e., "light," "low," or "mild," or similar descriptors by September 8, 2017, unless you have a Modified Risk Tobacco Product order in place.
- 2018
  - Include required warning statements on packages and advertisements on "covered" tobacco products (and roll-your-own/ cigarette tobacco products) by May 10, 2018.

*(Source: "Advertising And Promotion," U.S. Food and Drug Administration (FDA), November 2, 2016.)*

---

# Sponsoring An Event

Manufacturers, retailers, and distributors are restricted from sponsoring in a cigarette or smokeless brand name any athletic, musical, or other social or cultural event, or any entry or team in any event, per 21 CFR Part 1140.

# Use Of Brand Name, Logo, Symbol, Motto, And More

Manufacturers and distributors are prohibited from selling or distributing any item or service (other than cigarettes or smokeless tobacco or roll-your-own paper) that bears the brand name, logo, symbol, motto, etc., that are identifiable with those used for any brand of cigarettes or smokeless tobacco, per 21 CFR Part 1140.

# Free Sample Restrictions

The prohibition on the distribution of free samples applies to all "tobacco products," (except for smokeless tobacco products in a "qualified adult-only facility" and in limited quantities as specified in the law, per Section 102 of the Tobacco Control Act) including newly-deemed tobacco products—including their components and parts, but not accessories, per 21 CFR sect; 1140.16(d).

## What Is Considered A "Free Sample"?

If the prospective buyer lights and draws, puffs on, otherwise consumes the tobacco product, or leaves the retail establishment with a free tobacco product (in whole or part), this would constitute a "free sample" in violation of 21 CFR § 1140.16(d).

## What Is Not Considered A "Free Sample"?

Allowing prospective adult buyers to smell or handle one of the newly-deemed products is not considered distribution of a "free sample" as long as the product is not actually consumed, in whole or in part, in the retail facility for free and the prospective buyer does not leave the facility with a free tobacco product. In most circumstances, retail facilities, including vape shops, can allow customers to touch, hold, and smell their products without violating the free sample ban.

# Format And Display Requirements For Required Warning Statements On Advertisements

Advertisements include print advertisements and other advertisements with a visual component (including, for example, advertisements on signs, shelf-talkers, Web pages, and email). The required warning statement on advertisements must:

- Appear on the upper portion of the advertisement within the trim area;

- Occupy at least 20 percent of the area of the advertisement (warning area);

- Be printed in at least 12-point font size and ensure that the required warning statement occupies the greatest possible proportion of the warning area set aside for the required warning statement;

- Be printed in conspicuous and legible Helvetica bold or Arial bold type or other similar sans serif fonts and in black text on a white background or white text on a black background in a manner that contrasts by typography, layout, or color, with all other printed material on the advertisement;

- Be capitalized and punctuated;

- Be centered in the warning area in which the text is required to be printed and positioned such that the text of the required warning statement and the other textual information in the advertisement have the same orientation; and

- Be surrounded by a rectangular border that is the same color as the text of the required warning statement and that is not less than 3 millimeters (mm) or more than 4 mm.

# Chapter 10

# The Link Between Youth Smoking And Exposure To Smoking In Movies

- A "tobacco incident" is one occurrence of smoking or other tobacco use in a movie.

- "Incidents" are a measure of the number of occurrences of smoking or other tobacco use in a movie.

- A "tobacco impression" is one person seeing one incident.

- "Impressions" are a measure of total audience exposure.

- This report's movie sample comprises all movies that ranked among the top 10 in ticket sales ("top-grossing movies") in any week of their first-run release to U.S. Theaters.

## Overview

- Watching movies that include smoking causes young people to start smoking. The more smoking young people see on screen, the more likely they are to start smoking.

- The percentage of youth-rated movies (G, PG, PG-13) that were smokefree increased from 2002 to 2015 (from 35 percent to 62 percent). But in youth-rated movies that showed any smoking, the average number of tobacco incidents per movie climbed to historically high levels in 2014 [n=38] before returning to 2002 levels [n=20] in 2015.

---

About This Chapter: This chapter includes text excerpted from "Smoking In The Movies," Centers for Disease Control and Prevention (CDC), April 6, 2016.

- The Motion Picture Association of America (MPAA), the studios' organization that assigns ratings, provides a "smoking label" along with the regular rating for some movies that contain smoking. However, almost 9 of every 10 (89%) youth-rated, top-grossing movies with smoking do not carry an MPAA "smoking label."

- The 2012 Surgeon General's Report (Preventing Tobacco Use Among Youth and Young Adults) concluded that an industrywide standard to rate movies with tobacco incidents R could result in reductions in youth smoking.

- Giving an R rating to future movies with smoking would be expected to reduce the number of teen smokers by nearly 1 in 5 (18 percent) and prevent 1 million deaths from smoking among children alive today.

# Background

- In 2012, the Surgeon General concluded that exposure to onscreen smoking in movies causes young people to start smoking. Because of this exposure to smoking in movies:

  - 6.4 million children alive today will become smokers, and 2 million of these children will die prematurely from diseases caused by smoking.

- Between 2002 and 2015:

  - Almost half (46 percent) of top-grossing movies in the United States were rated PG-13.

  - 6 of every 10 PG-13 movies (59 percent) showed smoking or other tobacco use.

- All six major movie companies that belong to MPAA have published individual policies addressing tobacco depictions in their movies.

  - Disney (2004)

  - Time Warner's Warner Bros. (2005)

  - Comcast's Universal (2007)

  - Fox and Sony (2012)

  - Viacom's Paramount (2013)

# Additional 2015 Findings

- The percentage of PG-13 movies with tobacco incidents was virtually unchanged from 2014. [2014: 46%; 2015: 47%]

- About half of PG-13 movies (53%) remained tobacco-free in 2015—a level substantially unchanged since 2010 (57 percent tobacco-free).

- In 2015, the number of tobacco incidents in the average youth-rated movie with tobacco (20 incidents) was lower than in any year since 2009. The number in the average R-rated movie with tobacco (30 incidents) was lower than in any year since at least 2002.

- Movies rated G were tobacco-free for the fourth year in a row. However, the total number of tobacco incidents in movies rated PG more than tripled from 2014 to 2015 (from 27 to 88).

- PG-13 movies included fewer than half as many total tobacco incidents in 2015 (519) as they did in 2014 (1,165). The total number of incidents in youth-rated movies in 2015 (607) was approximately half the number in 2002 (1,296).

- The number of tobacco incidents in movies varies by movie company. From 2010 to 2015.

  - Tobacco incidents increased in youth-rated movies from independent movie companies, Disney, Fox, and Time Warner (Warner Bros.).

  - Tobacco incidents decreased in movies from Comcast (Universal), Sony, and Viacom (Paramount).

## Conclusions

- The data show that individual movie company policies alone have not been efficient at minimizing smoking in movies. Movie companies with tobacco depiction policies included tobacco in as many of their youth-rated movies in 2015 as they did in 2010 [18 in 2010; 19 in 2015] and each of these movies included nearly as many tobacco incidents, on average [25 incidents per movie in 2010; 22 incidents per movie in 2015].

- Reducing the number of tobacco incidents in movies will further protect young people from starting to use tobacco. Several strategies have been identified to reduce youth exposure to onscreen tobacco incidents:

  - The 2012 Surgeon General's Report concluded that an industrywide standard to rate movies with tobacco incidents R could result in reductions in youth smoking.

  - The 2014 Surgeon General's Report (*The Health Consequences of Smoking—50 Years of Progress*) concluded that youth rates of tobacco use would be reduced by 18 percent if tobacco incidents and impressions in PG-13 films were eliminated by such actions as having all future movies with tobacco incidents receive an R rating.

  - States and local jurisdictions could also work towards reducing tobacco incidents in movies.

# Chapter 11

# New Regulations For Tobacco Products

The U.S. Food and Drug Administration (FDA) recently finalized a rule that extends its regulatory authority to all tobacco products, including e-cigarettes, cigars, and hookah and pipe tobacco, as part of its goal to improve public health.

"Before this final rule, these products could be sold without any review of their ingredients, how they were made, and their potential dangers," explains Mitch Zeller, J.D., director of the U.S. Food and Drug Administration (FDA's) Center for Tobacco Products. "Under this new rule, we're taking steps to protect Americans from the dangers of tobacco products, ensure these tobacco products have health warnings, and restrict sales to minors."

## What Does This New Rule Do?

This new rule builds on groundwork that was set close to seven years ago. The FDA has regulated cigarettes, cigarette tobacco, roll-your-own tobacco, and smokeless tobacco products since June 2009, after Congress passed and the President signed the Family Smoking Prevention and Tobacco Control Act. This Act gave the agency authority to regulate the manufacturing, distribution, and marketing of tobacco products.

Today, the rule does several things.

It extends the FDA's regulatory authority to all tobacco products, including e-cigarettes—which are also called electronic cigarettes or electronic nicotine delivery systems (ENDS)—all cigars (including premium ones), hookah (also called waterpipe tobacco), pipe tobacco, nicotine gels, and dissolvables that did not previously fall under the FDA's authority.

About This Chapter: This chapter includes text excerpted from "The Facts On The FDA's New Tobacco Rule," U.S. Food and Drug Administration (FDA), June 16, 2016.

It requires health warnings on roll-your-own tobacco, cigarette tobacco, and certain newly regulated tobacco products and also bans free samples. In addition, because of the rule, manufacturers of newly regulated tobacco products that were not on the market as of February 15, 2007, will have to show that products meet the applicable public health standard set by the law. And those manufacturers will have to receive marketing authorization from the FDA.

The new rule also restricts youth access to newly regulated tobacco products by:

- not allowing products to be sold to those younger than 18 and requiring age verification via photo ID; and

- not allowing tobacco products to be sold in vending machines (unless in an adult-only facility).

Finally, it gives a foundation for future FDA actions related to tobacco.

## Why Did The FDA Take This Action?

The FDA's goal is to protect Americans from tobacco-related disease and death. Tobacco use is a major threat to public health.

It's important to note that FDA regulation of these products does not mean they are safe to use. But before this rule, there was no federal law to stop retailers from selling e-cigarettes, hookah, or cigars to youth under age 18. There has been a major drop in the use of traditional cigarettes among youth over the past decade, but their use of other tobacco products is rising. Current e-cigarette use among high school students has skyrocketed from 1.5 percent in 2011 to 16 percent in 2015 (a more than 900 percent increase) and hookah use has risen significantly, according to a survey supported by the FDA and the Centers for Disease Control and Prevention (CDC).

This rule allows the FDA to protect youth by restricting their access to tobacco products.

## What Product Characteristics Will The FDA Review?

The tobacco product review process allows the FDA to evaluate important factors such as ingredients, product design and health risks, as well as products' appeal to youth and non-users.

## What's The Timeline?

The FDA expects that manufacturers will continue selling their products for up to two years while they submit—and an additional year while the FDA reviews—a new tobacco product application.

The FDA will issue an order to give marketing authorization where appropriate. Otherwise, the product will face FDA enforcement.

## What's The Bottom Line?

The rule will help prevent young people from starting to use these products, help consumers better understand the risks of using these products, prohibit false and misleading product claims, and prevent new tobacco products from being marketed unless a manufacturer demonstrates that the products meet the relevant public health standard.

## But Aren't E-Cigarettes Safer Than Regular Cigarettes? And What About The Burden On Small Businesses?

The FDA recognizes that some tobacco products have the potential to be less harmful than others. But more evidence is needed. The agency is exploring this issue with respect to tobacco regulation.

The FDA believes that this new technology has both potential benefits and risks. If certain products, such as e-cigarettes, have reduced toxicity compared to conventional cigarettes; encourage current smokers to switch completely; and/or are not widely used by youth, they may have the potential to reduce disease and death. But if any product prompts young people to become addicted to nicotine, reduces a person's interest in quitting cigarettes, and/or leads to long-term usage with other tobacco products, the public health impact could be negative.

The FDA encourages manufacturers to explore product innovations that would maximize potential benefits and minimize risks. The final rule allows the FDA to further evaluate and assess the impact of these products on the health of both users and non-users. And it lets the FDA regulate the products based on the most current scientific knowledge.

The FDA considered all manufacturers, including small businesses, when finalizing this rule. That's why the agency is allowing additional time for small-scale tobacco product manufacturers to comply with certain provisions.

# So Which Products Can Help Me Quit Using Tobacco?

The FDA has approved a variety of products as cessation aids to help reduce your dependence on nicotine. Products include nicotine gum, nicotine skin patches, nicotine lozenges, nicotine oral inhaled products, and nicotine nasal spray as well as non-nicotine medications called varenicline and bupropion.

# Chapter 12

# Selected Actions Of The U.S. Government Regarding The Regulation Of Tobacco

## About Tobacco Laws And Regulations

### Why Is Tobacco Control Important?

Tobacco control programs aim to reduce disease, disability, and death related to tobacco use. A comprehensive approach—one that includes educational, clinical, regulatory, economic, and social strategies—has been established as the best way to eliminate the negative health and economic effects of tobacco use.

### What Is The Difference Between A Law And A Regulation?

Federal laws, like the Family Smoking Prevention and Tobacco Control Act (Tobacco Control Act), are passed by Congress and signed by the president. These laws are usually enforced through executive branch agencies, such as the U.S. Food and Drug Administration (FDA).

Laws can also be enacted at the state and local level to protect public health and make tobacco products less affordable, less accessible, and less attractive. For example, states may pass smokefree indoor air laws and cigarette price increases, which have been proven to reduce cigarette use, prevent youth from starting to smoke, and encourage people to try to quit.

---

About This Chapter: Text under the heading "About Tobacco Laws And Regulations" is excerpted from "Laws/Policies," BeTobaccoFree.gov, U.S. Department of Health and Human Services (HHS), November 15, 2012. Reviewed December 2016; Text under the heading "Selected Actions Of The U.S. Government" is excerpted from "Smoking And Tobacco Use," Centers for Disease Control and Prevention (CDC), July 28, 2015.

The executive branch, when authorized by Congress, enacts Federal regulations. States can also introduce regulations. Most regulations are developed by a government agency with public input. For example, FDA issues tobacco-related regulations under authority provided by the Tobacco Control Act through a notice and comment rulemaking process. This process allows for public input before FDA issues the final regulation.

# Selected Actions Of The U.S. Government

## Food and Drugs Act of 1906

- First federal food and drug law

- No express reference to tobacco products

- Definition of a drug includes medicines and preparations listed in U.S. Pharmacoepia or National Formulary.

- 1914 interpretation advised that tobacco be included only when used to cure, mitigate, or prevent disease.

## Federal Food, Drug, and Cosmetic Act (FFDCA) of 1938

- Superseded 1906 Act

- Definition of a "drug" includes "articles intended for use in the diagnosis, cure, mitigation, treatment, or prevention of disease in man or other animals" and "articles (other than food) intended to affect the structure or any function of the body of man or other animals".

- FDA has asserted jurisdiction in cases where the manufacturer or vendor has made medical claims.

    - 1953—Fairfax cigarettes (manufacturer claimed these prevented respiratory and other diseases)

    - 1959—Trim Reducing-Aid Cigarettes (contained the additive tartaric acid, which was claimed to aid in weight reduction)

- FDA has asserted jurisdiction over alternative nicotine-delivery products

    - 1984—Nicotine Polacrilex gum

    - 1985—Favor Smokeless Cigarette (nicotine-delivery device; ruled a "new drug," intended to treat nicotine dependence and to affect the structure and function of the body; removed from market)

- 1989—Masterpiece Tobacs tobacco chewing gum; ruled an adulterated food and removed from the market)
- 1991—Nicotine patches

## Federal Trade Commission (FTC) Act of 1914 (amended in 1938)

- Empowers the FTC to "prevent persons, partnerships, or corporations ... from using unfair or deceptive acts or practices in commerce."

- Between 1945 and 1960, FTC completed seven formal cease-and-desist order proceedings for medical or health claims (e.g., a 1942 complaint countering claims that Kool cigarettes provide extra protection against or cure colds).

- In January 1964, FTC proposed a rule to strictly regulate the imagery and copy of cigarette ads to prohibit explicit or implicit health claims.

- 1983—FTC determines that its testing procedures may have "significantly underestimated the level of tar, nicotine, and carbon monoxide that smokers received from smoking" certain low-tar cigarettes. Prohibits Brown and Williamson Tobacco Company from using the tar rating for Barclay cigarettes in advertising, packaging or promotions because of problems with the testing methodology and consumers' possible reliance on that information. FTC authorized revised labeling in 1986.

- 1985—FTC acts to remove the RJ Reynolds advertisements, "Of Cigarettes and Science," in which the multiple risk factor intervention trail (MRFIT) results were misinterpreted.

- 1999—FTC requires RJ Reynolds to add a label to packages and ads explaining that "no additives" does not make Winston cigarettes safer.

## Federal Hazardous Substances Labeling Act (FHSA) of 1960

- Authorized FDA to regulate substances that are hazardous (either toxic, corrosive, irritant, strong sensitizers, flammable, or pressure-generating). Such substances may cause substantial personal injury or illness during or as a result of customary use.

- 1963—FDA expressed its interpretation that tobacco did not fit the "hazardous" criteria stated previously and withheld recommendations pending the release of the report of the Surgeon General's Advisory Committee on Smoking and Health.

## Federal Cigarette Labeling and Advertising Act of 1965

- Required package warning label—"Caution: Cigarette Smoking May Be Hazardous to Your Health" (other health warnings prohibited).

- Required no labels on cigarette advertisements (in fact, implemented a three-year prohibition of any such labels).

- Required FTC to report to Congress annually on the effectiveness of cigarette labeling, current cigarette advertising and promotion practices, and to make recommendations for legislation.

- Required Department of Health, Education, and Welfare (DHEW) to report annually to Congress on the health consequences of smoking.

## Public Health Cigarette Smoking Act of 1969

- Required package warning label—"Warning: The Surgeon General Has Determined that Cigarette Smoking Is Dangerous to Your Health" (other health warnings prohibited).

- Temporarily preempted FTC requirement of health labels on advertisements.

- Prohibited cigarette advertising on television and radio (authority to U.S. Department of Justice [DOJ]).

- Prevents states or localities from regulating or prohibiting cigarette advertising or promotion for health-related reasons.

## Controlled Substances Act of 1970

- To prevent the abuse of drugs, narcotics, and other addictive substances.

- Specifically excludes tobacco from the definition of a "controlled substance."

## Consumer Product Safety Act of 1972

- Transferred authority from the FDA to regulate hazardous substances as designated by the Federal Hazardous Substances Labeling Act (FHSA) to the Consumer Product Safety Commission (CPSC).

- The term "consumer product" does not include tobacco and tobacco products.

## Little Cigar Act of 1973

- Bans little cigar advertisements from television and radio (authority to DOJ)

## 1976 Amendment to the Federal Hazardous Substances Labeling Act of 1960

- The term "hazardous substance" shall not apply to tobacco and tobacco products (passed when the American Public Health Association petitioned CPSC to set a maximum level of 21 mg. of tar in cigarettes)

## Toxic Substances Control Act of 1976

- To "regulate chemical substances and mixtures which present an unreasonable risk of injury to health or the environment."

- The term "chemical substance" does not include tobacco or any tobacco products.

## Comprehensive Smoking Education Act of 1984

- Requires four rotating health warning labels (all listed as Surgeon General's Warnings) on cigarette packages and advertisements (smoking causes lung cancer, heart disease and may complicate pregnancy; quitting smoking now greatly reduces serious risks to your health; smoking by pregnant women may result in fetal injury, premature birth, and low birth weight; cigarette smoke contains carbon monoxide) (preempted other package warnings).

- Requires Department of Health and Human Services (DHHS) to publish a biennial status report to Congress on smoking and health.

- Creates a Federal Interagency Committee on Smoking and Health.

- Requires cigarette industry to provide a confidential list of ingredients added to cigarettes manufactured in or imported into the United States (brand-specific ingredients and quantities not required).

## Cigarette Safety Act of 1984

- To determine the technical and commercial feasibility of developing cigarettes and little cigars that would be less likely to ignite upholstered furniture and mattresses

## Comprehensive Smokeless Tobacco Health Education Act of 1986

- Institutes three rotating health warning labels on smokeless tobacco packages and advertisements (this product may cause mouth cancer; this product may cause gum disease

63

and tooth loss; this product is not a safe alternative to cigarettes) (preempts other health warnings on packages or advertisements [except billboards]).

- Prohibits smokeless tobacco advertising on television and radio.

- Requires DHHS to publish a biennial status report to Congress on smokeless tobacco.

- Requires FTC to report to Congress on smokeless tobacco sales, advertising, and marketing.

- Requires smokeless tobacco companies to provide a confidential list of additives and a specification of nicotine content in smokeless tobacco products.

- Requires DHHS to conduct public information campaign on the health hazards of smokeless tobacco.

## Public Law 100-202 (1987)

- Banned smoking on domestic airline flights scheduled for two hours or less.

## Public Law 101-164 (1989)

- Bans smoking on domestic airline flights scheduled for six hours or less.

## Synar Amendment to the Alcohol, Drug Abuse, and Mental Health Administration (ADAMHA) Reorganization Act of 1992

- Requires all states to adopt and enforce restrictions on tobacco sales and distribution to minors.

## Pro-Children Act of 1994

- Requires all federally funded children's services to become smokefree. Expands upon 1993 law that banned smoking in Women, Infants, and Children (WIC) clinics.

## Family Smoking Prevention and Tobacco Control Act of 2009

- Grants the U.S. Food and Drug Administration (FDA) the authority to regulate tobacco products.

# Part Two
## Nicotine Delivery Systems

# Chapter 13
# Cigarettes And Brand Preferences

## Cigarettes

### Market Share Information (United States)

- According to 2015 sales data, Marlboro is the most popular cigarette brand in the United States, with sales greater than the next four leading competitors combined.

- The three most heavily advertised brands—Marlboro, Newport, and Camel—continue to be the preferred brands of cigarettes smoked by young people.

**Table 13.1.** 2015 Market Shares For Leading Cigarette Brands

| Brand | Market % |
|---|---|
| Marlboro | 41% |
| Newport | 13% |
| Camel (filter only) | 8% |
| Pall Mall Box | 8% |
| Pyramid | 2% |
| Maverick | 2% |
| Santa Fe | 2% |
| Winston | 2% |
| Kool | 2% |

NOTE: Market share—or market percentage—is defined as the percentage of total sales in the United States.

---

About This Chapter: This chapter includes text excerpted from "Tobacco Brand Preferences," Centers for Disease Control and Prevention (CDC), December 1, 2016.

## Industry Marketing Practices

Tobacco industry marketing practices can influence the brands that certain groups prefer. For example:

- The packaging and design of certain cigarette brands appeal to adolescents and young adults.

- Historically, menthol cigarettes have been targeted heavily toward certain racial/ethnic groups, especially African Americans.

  - Among African American adult, adolescent, and young adult cigarette smokers, the most popular brands are all mentholated.

- Cigarettes with brand names containing words such as "thins" and "slims" have been manufactured to be longer and slimmer than traditional cigarettes to appeal directly to women—e.g., Virginia Slims and Capri brands.

## Brand Characteristics

- Of all the cigarettes sold in the United States in 2013—

  - 99.7 percent were filtered

  - 31 percent were mentholated brands

- Use of mentholated brands varies widely by race/ethnicity. The percentage of individuals aged 12 years or older who reported using mentholated brands in 2010 was:

  - 19.1 percent Black

  - 3.6 percent Asian

  - 7.8 percent Hispanic

  - 6.5 percent White

- Before 2010, manufacturers were allowed to label cigarettes as "light" or "ultra light" if they delivered less than 15 mg of tar when measured by an automated smoking machine.

  - Such labeling allowed tobacco companies to deliberately misrepresent "light" cigarettes as being less harmful and an acceptable alternative to quitting smoking.

  - The 2009 Family Smoking Prevention and Tobacco Control Act, however, prohibited use of terms like "light," "low," and "mild" on tobacco product labels.

# Chapter 14
# "Light" Cigarettes

## What Is A So-Called Light Cigarette?

Tobacco manufacturers have been redesigning cigarettes since the 1950s. Certain redesigned cigarettes with the following features were marketed as "light" cigarettes:

- Cellulose acetate filters (to trap tar).

- Highly porous cigarette paper (to allow toxic chemicals to escape).

- Ventilation holes in the filter tip (to dilute smoke with air).

- Different blends of tobacco.

When analyzed by a smoking machine, the smoke from a so-called light cigarette has a lower yield of tar than the smoke from a regular cigarette. However, a machine cannot predict how much tar a smoker inhales. Also, studies have shown that changes in cigarette design have not lowered the risk of disease caused by cigarettes.

On June 22, 2009, President Barack Obama signed into law the Family Smoking Prevention and Tobacco Control Act, which granted the U.S. Food and Drug Administration (FDA) the authority to regulate tobacco products. One provision of the new law bans tobacco manufacturers from using the terms "light," "low," and "mild" in product labeling and advertisements. This provision went into effect on June 22, 2010. However, some tobacco manufacturers are using color-coded packaging (such as gold or silver packaging) on previously marketed products and selling them to consumers who may continue to believe that these cigarettes are not as harmful as other cigarettes.

About This Chapter: This chapter includes text excerpted from ""Light" Cigarettes And Cancer Risk," National Cancer Institute (NCI), October 28, 2010. Reviewed December 2016.

# Are Light Cigarettes Less Hazardous Than Regular Cigarettes?

No. Many smokers chose so-called low-tar, mild, light, or ultralight cigarettes because they thought these cigarettes would expose them to less tar and would be less harmful to their health than regular or full-flavor cigarettes. However, light cigarettes are no safer than regular cigarettes. Tar exposure from a light cigarette can be just as high as that from a regular cigarette if the smoker takes long, deep, or frequent puffs. The bottom line is that light cigarettes do not reduce the health risks of smoking.

Moreover, there is no such thing as a safe cigarette. The only guaranteed way to reduce the risk to your health, as well as the risk to others, is to stop smoking completely.

Because all tobacco products are harmful and cause cancer, the use of these products is strongly discouraged. There is no safe level of tobacco use. People who use any type of tobacco product should quit.

# Do Light Cigarettes Cause Cancer?

Yes. People who smoke any kind of cigarette are at much greater risk of lung cancer than people who do not smoke. Smoking harms nearly every organ of the body and diminishes a person's overall health.

People who switched to light cigarettes from regular cigarettes are likely to have inhaled the same amount of toxic chemicals, and they remain at high risk of developing smoking-related cancers and other disease. Smoking causes cancers of the lung, esophagus, larynx (voice box), mouth, throat, kidney, bladder, pancreas, stomach, and cervix, as well as acute myeloid leukemia.

Regardless of their age, smokers can substantially reduce their risk of disease, including cancer, by quitting.

# What Were The Tar Yield Ratings Used By The Tobacco Industry For Light Cigarettes?

Although no Federal agency formally defined the range of tar yield for light or ultralight cigarettes, the tobacco industry used the ranges shown in the table 14.1 below.

**Table 14.1.** Tar In Light Cigarettes

| Industry Terms on Packages | Machine-measured Tar Yield (in milligrams) |
| --- | --- |
| Ultralight or Ultralow tar | Usually 7 or less |
| Light or Low tar | Usually 8–14 |
| Full flavor or Regular | Usually 15 or more |

These ratings were not an accurate indicator of how much tar a smoker might have been exposed to, because people do not smoke cigarettes the same way the machines do and no two people smoke the same way.

Ultralight and light cigarettes are no safer than full-flavor cigarettes. There is no such thing as a safe cigarette.

## Are Machine-Measured Tar Yields Misleading?

Yes. The ratings cannot be used to predict how much tar a smoker will actually get because the way the machine smokes a cigarette is not the way a person smokes a cigarette. A rating of 7 milligrams does not mean that you will get only 7 milligrams of tar. You can get just as much tar from a light cigarette as from a full-flavor cigarette. It all depends on how you smoke. Taking deeper, longer, and more frequent puffs will lead to greater tar exposure. Also, a smoker's lips or fingers may block the air ventilation holes in the filter, leading to greater tar exposure.

## Why Would Someone Smoking A Light Cigarette Take Bigger Puffs Than With A Regular Cigarette?

Cigarette features that reduce the yield of machine-measured tar also reduce the yield of nicotine. Because smokers crave nicotine, they may inhale more deeply; take larger, more rapid, or more frequent puffs; or smoke extra cigarettes each day to get enough nicotine to satisfy their craving. As a result, smokers end up inhaling more tar, nicotine, and other harmful chemicals than the machine-based numbers suggest.

Tobacco industry documents show that companies were aware that smokers of light cigarettes compensated by taking bigger puffs. Industry documents also show that the companies were aware of the difference between machine-measured yields of tar and nicotine and what the smoker actually inhaled.

# Chapter 15
# Menthol Cigarettes

## What Are Menthol Cigarettes?

Menthol is a substance naturally found in mint plants such as peppermint and spearmint. It gives a cooling sensation. It is often used to relieve minor pain and irritation and prevent infection.

Menthol is added to many products. These include lozenges, syrups, creams and ointments, nasal sprays, powders, and candy. But none of these products are lighted or smoked when used. That makes them different from menthol cigarettes.

Many smokers think menthol cigarettes are less harmful. There is no evidence that cigarettes, cigars, or smokeless tobacco products that have menthol are safer than other cigarettes.

Like other cigarettes, menthol cigarettes harm nearly every organ in the body. They cause many diseases, including cancer and heart disease. Some research shows that menthol cigarettes may be more addictive than non-menthol cigarettes.

## Menthol Marketing

Menthol was first added to cigarettes in the 1920s. In the past, the tobacco industry marketed menthol cigarettes as being healthier and safer. Advertisements emphasized their cool

About This Chapter: Text beginning with the heading "Menthol Cigarettes" is excerpted from "Know More About Menthol Cigarettes," Smokefree.gov, U.S. Department of Health and Human Services (HHS), June 5, 2016; Text under the heading "Menthol Cigarettes And Health Concerns" is excerpted from "FDA Invites Public Input On Menthol In Cigarettes," U.S. Food and Drug Administration (FDA), July 23, 2013. Reviewed December 2016; Text under the heading "FAQs About Menthol Cigarettes" is excerpted from "Menthol Cigarettes," Smokefree.gov, U.S. Department of Health and Human Services (HHS), February 12, 2010. Reviewed December 2016.

and refreshing taste. The ads often showed nature, coldness, springtime, water, and other refreshing qualities. The tobacco industry also targeted "beginner" smokers, smokers with health concerns, and certain population groups. Many people chose menthol cigarettes because they believed they were safer than non-menthol cigarettes. They are not.

# Menthol Cigarettes And Health Concerns

"Menthol cigarettes raise critical public health questions," said U.S. Food and Drug Administration (FDA) Commissioner Margaret A. Hamburg, M.D. "The FDA is committed to a science-based approach that addresses the public health issues raised by menthol cigarettes, and public input will help us make more informed decisions about how best to tackle this important issue moving forward."

The agency is issuing the Advance Notice of Proposed Rulemaking (ANPRM) to obtain additional information related to potential regulatory options it might consider, such as establishing tobacco product standards, among others.

The ANPRM will be available for public comment for 60 days. The FDA will consider all comments, data, research, and other information submitted to the docket to determine what, if any, regulatory action with respect to menthol in cigarettes is appropriate. If the FDA decides to issue a rule, the first step in that process would be a Notice of Proposed Rulemaking, which would give the public an opportunity to weigh in on the specifics of the proposed rule.

"FDA's actions today on menthol reflect our commitment to explore all potential options, including the establishment of product standards. In the meantime, we will conduct new research to further inform our decision making," said Mitch Zeller, J.D., director of the FDA's Center for Tobacco Products.

The agency is also making available for public comment relevant scientific information, including the FDA's independent Preliminary Scientific Evaluation of the Possible Public Health Effects of Menthol Versus Nonmenthol Cigarettes. The preliminary evaluation addresses the association between menthol cigarettes and various outcomes, including initiation, addiction, and cessation.

In addition, the FDA plans to support new research on the differences between menthol and nonmenthol cigarettes as they relate to menthol's likely impact on smoking cessation and attempts to quit, as well as assessing the levels of menthol in cigarette brands and sub-brands. The FDA is funding three menthol-related studies; one to look at whether genetic differences in taste perceptions explain why certain racial and ethnic populations are more likely to use menthol cigarettes; the second to compare exposure to smoke-related toxins and carcinogens from menthol and nonmenthol cigarettes; and a third to examine the effects of menthol and nonmenthol compounds in various tobacco products on both tobacco addiction and toxicants of tobacco smoke.

Finally, the FDA is developing a youth education campaign focused on preventing and reducing tobacco use, including menthol cigarettes.

# FAQs About Menthol Cigarettes

## What Is Menthol?

Menthol is a substance naturally found in mint plants such as peppermint and spearmint. It gives a cooling sensation and is frequently used to relieve minor pain and irritation and to prevent infection.

## Which Tobacco Products Contain Menthol?

Menthol is found in cigarettes, cigars, little cigars, smokeless tobacco products, and tobacco rolling paper.

## How Much Menthol Is Found In Cigarettes?

Only cigarettes containing a certain amount of menthol (0.1% to 0.45% of the tobacco filler weight) are marketed and advertised as menthol cigarettes.

> About 90 percent of cigarettes marketed in the United States contain menthol, even if they are not advertised as menthol cigarettes.

## What Are Some Common Menthol Cigarette Brands?

Some common cigarette brands that are only made in menthol flavor include Kool, Newport, and Salem. Other brands of menthol and non-menthol cigarettes include Doral, Virginia Slims, Marlboro, and Camel.

Of all menthol and non-menthol cigarettes, Marlboro is the brand used most often by 42.2 percent of smokers. Newport is second (11.3%), followed by Camel (7.5%), Basic (4.2%), Doral (3.1%), Kool (2.9%), Parliament (2%), Salem (1.9%), and USA Gold (1.9%).

## What Is The Difference Between Menthol And Non-Menthol Cigarettes?

Aside from the amount of menthol added, we need more research to understand the main differences between these cigarette types and how they are harmful to your health.

## Is It Safer To Smoke A Menthol Cigarette Than A Non-Menthol Cigarette?

No. All cigarettes are harmful, including menthol cigarettes. Many smokers think menthol cigarettes are less harmful, but there is no evidence that menthol cigarettes are safer than other cigarettes. Like other cigarettes, menthol cigarettes harm nearly every organ in the body and cause many diseases, including cancer, cardiovascular diseases, and respiratory diseases. Menthol cigarettes, like other cigarettes, also negatively impact male and female fertility and are harmful to pregnant women and their unborn babies.

## Do Menthol Cigarettes Contain Fiberglass?

There is no evidence to suggest that fiberglass (used to make car parts) is in menthol cigarettes. However, there are more than 7,000 known chemical compounds, as well as toxic and carcinogenic agents, in tobacco and cigarette smoke. Some of these include ammonia (used in fertilizer and household cleaning products), formaldehyde (used to preserve dead bodies), and methanol (used in antifreeze). All of these chemicals have been shown to cause cancer and other deadly diseases.

## Are Menthol Cigarettes More Addictive Than Non-Menthol Cigarettes?

More research is needed to understand how addiction differs between menthol and non-menthol cigarette use.

> Some research shows that menthol cigarettes may be more addictive than non-menthol cigarettes.

## Why Do People Smoke Menthol Cigarettes?

In the past, the tobacco industry has marketed menthol cigarettes as being a "healthier" and "safer" cigarette, emphasizing its cool and refreshing taste. The tobacco industry has targeted "beginner" smokers and current smokers with health concerns. Many people choose menthol cigarettes because of beliefs about menthol cigarettes being safer than non-menthol cigarettes. However, no evidence exists indicating that menthol cigarettes are safer. All cigarette smoking is linked to many cancers and other diseases.

## How Has The Tobacco Industry Marketed And Encouraged People To Smoke Menthol Cigarettes?

In the past, the tobacco industry has actively marketed menthol cigarettes to consumers under a concept of "coolness," with messages of fresh/refreshing taste and sensation, youthfulness, fun, and healthful effects. Advertisements often showed nature, coldness, springtime, water, and other refreshing qualities.

## Does The Tobacco Industry Market Menthol Cigarettes To Anyone In Particular?

Yes. Studies and evidence from tobacco industry documents showed that, in the past, the tobacco industry has a history of marketing menthol cigarettes to women, youth, and minority racial/ethnic groups, including African Americans/Blacks, Latinos/Hispanics, and Asian Americans.

Research suggests that African American/Blacks may be the most directly targeted group of menthol smokers.

## Is Menthol In Other Products?

Yes. Menthol is added to many other products, including:

- Candy
- Creams/ointments
- Lozenges
- Nasal sprays
- Powders
- Syrups

Menthol is generally used in small amounts to temporarily relieve throat irritations and coughs from colds or inhaled irritants. But keep in mind that none of these products are ignited or smoked when used.

# Chapter 16
# Electronic Cigarettes

Electronic cigarettes (also called e-cigarettes or electronic nicotine delivery systems) are battery-operated devices designed to deliver nicotine with flavorings and other chemicals to users in vapor instead of smoke. They can be manufactured to resemble traditional tobacco cigarettes, cigars or pipes, or even everyday items like pens or USB memory sticks; newer devices, such as those with fillable tanks, may look different. More than 250 different e-cigarette brands are currently on the market.

About 69% of middle and high school students were exposed to e-cigarette advertisements in retail stores, on the Internet, in magazines/newspapers, or on TV/movies. Exposure to e-cigarette advertisements may be contributing to increases in e-cigarette use among youth.

*(Source: "E-Cigarette Ads And Youth," Centers for Disease Control and Prevention (CDC), January 5, 2016.)*

While e-cigarettes are often promoted as safer alternatives to traditional cigarettes, which deliver nicotine by burning tobacco, little is actually known yet about the health risks of using these devices.

---

About This Chapter: This chapter includes text excerpted from "DrugFacts—Electronic Cigarettes (E-Cigarettes)," National Institute on Drug Abuse (NIDA), May 2016.

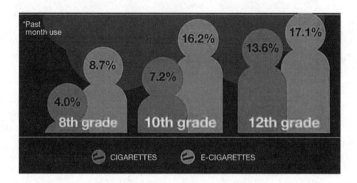

**Figure 16.1.** Teens Are More Likely To Use E-Cigarettes Than Cigarettes

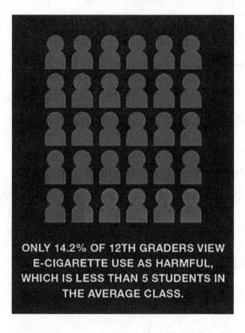

**Figure 16.2.** 12th Graders View Of E-Cigarettes

*(Source: "Knowns And Unknowns About E-Cigarettes And Teens," National Institute on Drug Abuse (NIDA), February 3, 2015.)*

# How Do E-Cigarettes Work?

Most e-cigarettes consist of three different components, including:

- a cartridge, which holds a liquid solution containing varying amounts of nicotine, flavorings, and other chemicals

- a heating device (vaporizer)

- a power source (usually a battery)

In many e-cigarettes, puffing activates the battery-powered heating device, which vaporizes the liquid in the cartridge. The resulting aerosol or vapor is then inhaled (called "vaping").

## Are E-Cigarettes Safer Than Conventional Cigarettes?

Unfortunately, this question is difficult to answer because insufficient information is available on these new products.

Cigarette smoking remains the leading preventable cause of sickness and mortality, responsible for over 400,000 deaths in the United States each year. The worst health consequences associated with smoking (e.g., cancer and heart disease) are linked to inhalation of tar and other chemicals produced by tobacco combustion; the pleasurable, reinforcing, and addictive properties of smoking are produced mostly by the nicotine contained in tobacco.

E-cigarettes are designed to simulate the act of tobacco smoking by producing an appealingly flavored aerosol that looks and feels like tobacco smoke and delivers nicotine but with less of the toxic chemicals produced by burning tobacco leaves. Because they deliver nicotine without burning tobacco, e-cigarettes appear as if they may be a safer, less toxic alternative to conventional cigarettes.

Although they do not produce tobacco smoke, e-cigarettes still contain nicotine and other potentially harmful chemicals. Nicotine is a highly addictive drug, and recent research suggests nicotine exposure may also prime the brain to become addicted to other substances. Also, testing of some e-cigarette products found the vapor to contain known carcinogens and toxic chemicals (such as formaldehyde and acetaldehyde), as well as potentially toxic metal nanoparticles from the vaporizing mechanism. The health consequences of repeated exposure to these chemicals are not yet clear.

Another worry is the refillable cartridges used by some e-cigarettes. Users may expose themselves to potentially toxic levels of nicotine when refilling them. Cartridges could also be filled with substances other than nicotine, thus possibly serving as a new and potentially dangerous way to deliver other drugs.

## Can E-Cigarettes Help A Person Quit Smoking?

Some people believe e-cigarette products may help smokers lower nicotine cravings while they are trying to discontinue their tobacco use. However, at this point it is unclear whether e-cigarettes may be effective as smoking-cessation aids. There is also the possibility that they could perpetuate the nicotine addiction and thus interfere with quitting.

These products have not been thoroughly evaluated in scientific studies. This may change in the near future, but for now, very little data exists on the safety of e-cigarettes, and consumers have no way of knowing whether there are any therapeutic benefits or how the health effects compare to conventional cigarettes.

## E-Cigarette Use By Youth

E-Cigarettes are increasingly popular among teens. Some states have banned sale of e-cigarettes to minors, but teens have been ordering them online. Their easy availability (online or via mall kiosks), in addition to their wide array of cartridge flavors (such as coffee, mint, candy, and fruit flavors), have helped make them particularly appealing to this age group. As a part of the FDA's new regulation to protect the health of our youth, minors will no longer be able to buy e-cigarettes in person or online.

In addition to the unknown health effects, early evidence suggests that e-cigarette use may serve as an introductory product for youth who then go on to use other tobacco products, including conventional cigarettes, which are known to cause disease and lead to premature death. A recent study showed that students who have used e-cigarettes by the time they start 9th grade are more likely than others to start smoking traditional cigarettes and other smokable tobacco products within the next year.

# Chapter 17

# Bidis And Kreteks

- Bidis are small, thin, hand-rolled cigarettes imported to the United States, primarily from India and other Southeast Asian countries. They comprise tobacco wrapped in a tendu or temburni leaf (plants native to Asia) and may be secured with a colorful string at one or both ends. Bidis can be flavored (e.g., chocolate, cherry, mango) or unflavored.

- Kreteks—sometimes referred to as clove cigarettes—are imported from Indonesia and typically contain a mixture of tobacco, cloves, and other additives.

- Bidis and kreteks have higher concentrations of nicotine, tar, and carbon monoxide than conventional cigarettes sold in the United States.

- Neither bidis nor kreteks are safe alternatives to conventional cigarettes.

## Health Effects

### Bidis

Because of the low prevalence of use, a limited amount of research on the long-term health effects of bidis has been conducted in the United States. However, research studies from India indicate that bidi smoking is associated with cancer and other adverse health conditions.

- Bidis are a combustible tobacco product. Smoke from a bidi contains three to five times the amount of nicotine as a regular cigarette and places users at risk for nicotine addiction.

---

About This Chapter: This chapter includes text excerpted from "Bidis And Kreteks," Centers for Disease Control and Prevention (CDC), February 22, 2016.

- Bidi smoking increases the risk for oral cancer, lung cancer, stomach cancer, and esophageal cancer.

- Bidi smoking is associated with a more than threefold increased risk for coronary heart disease and acute myocardial infarction (heart attack).

- Bidi smoking is associated with emphysema and a nearly fourfold increased risk for chronic bronchitis.

## Kreteks

Because of the low prevalence of use, a limited amount of research on the long-term health effects of kreteks has been conducted in the United States. However, research studies from Indonesia indicate that kretek smoking is associated with lung problems.

- Kretek smoking is associated with an increased risk for acute lung injury (i.e., lung damage that can include a range of characteristics, such as decreased oxygen, fluid in the lungs, leakage from capillaries, and inflammation), especially among susceptible individuals with asthma or respiratory infections.

- Regular kretek smokers have 13 to 20 times the risk for abnormal lung function (e.g., airflow obstruction or reduced oxygen absorption) compared with nonsmokers.

# Current Estimates

## Bidis

Percentage of U.S. students who were current bidi smokers* in 2014

- 0.5 percent of all middle school students

- 0.3 percent of female middle school students†

- 0.9 percent of all high school students

- 0.6 percent of female high school students

- 1.2 percent of male high school students

*Current smokers are defined as persons who reported smoking 1 or more bidis or kreteks in the 30 days before they participated in a survey about this topic.*

*† Data for middle school males are statistically unreliable as sample size was <50 or relative standard error was >0.3; therefore an estimate is not provided.*

## Kreteks

- The Family Smoking Prevention and Tobacco Control Act (Tobacco Control Act) of 2009 prohibits the sale of flavored cigarettes in the United States; therefore, data on the use of kreteks are no longer collected.

# Chapter 18

# Cigars

- A cigar is defined as a roll of tobacco wrapped in leaf tobacco or in a substance that contains tobacco.

- Cigars differ from cigarettes in that cigarettes are a roll of tobacco wrapped in paper or in a substance that does not contain tobacco.

- The three major types of cigars sold in the United States are large cigars, cigarillos, and little cigars.

- The use of flavorings in some cigar brands and the fact that they are commonly sold as a single stick has raised concerns that these products may be especially appealing to youth.

- In 2014, among middle and high school students who used cigars in the past 30 days, 63.5 percent reported using a flavored cigar during that time.

- Little cigars are the same size and shape as cigarettes, often include a filter, and are packaged in a similar way, but they are taxed differently than cigarettes. Rather than reduce consumption, cost-conscious smokers might switch from cigarettes to less costly little cigars.

- Historically, cigar smoking in the United States has been a behavior of older men, but the industry's increased marketing of these products to targeted groups in the 1990s increased the prevalence of use among adolescents.

- Cigar use is higher among youth who use other tobacco products or other drugs (e.g., alcohol, marijuana, and inhalants) than among youth who do not use these products.

About This Chapter: This chapter includes text excerpted from "Cigars," Centers for Disease Control and Prevention (CDC), February 22, 2016.

**Table 18.1.** Description And Market Share Of Cigar Types

| Type | Description | Market Share (2014)* |
|------|-------------|----------------------|
| Large cigar | Cigar that typically contains at least one-half ounce of aged, fermented tobacco (i.e., as much as a pack of cigarettes) and usually takes 1 to 2 hours to smoke | 96% |
| Cigarillo | A short (3–4 inches) and narrow cigar that typically contains about 3 grams of tobacco and usually does not include a filter | |
| Little cigar | A small cigar that typically is about the same size as a cigarette and usually includes a filter | 4% |

*\* Percentage of U.S. market for cigar products. Large cigar and cigarillo categories are combined in the calculation of market share.*

# Health Effects

- Regular cigar smoking is associated with an increased risk for cancers of the lung, esophagus, larynx (voice box), and oral cavity (lip, tongue, mouth, throat).

- Cigar smoking is linked to gum disease and tooth loss.

- Heavy cigar smokers and those who inhale deeply may be at increased risk for developing coronary heart disease.

- Heavy cigar smoking increases the risk for lung diseases, such as emphysema and chronic bronchitis.

> Cigars contain the same toxic and carcinogenic compounds found in cigarettes and are not a safe alternative to cigarettes.

# Current Cigar Use

## Adults*

Percentage of U.S. adults who were current cigar smokers† in 2013:

- 5 percent of all adults

- 8.2 percent of adult males

- 2 percent of adult females

- 7.5 percent of African American adults

- 6.7 percent of American Indian/Alaska Native adults

- 2.1 percent of Asian American adults

- 4 percent of Hispanic adults

- 5 percent of White adults

## High School Students

Percentage of U.S. high school students who were current smokers† in 2014:

- 8.2 percent of all students in grades 9–12

- 5.5 percent of female students in grades 9–12

- 10.8 percent of male students in grades 9–12

- Cigar use among high school males (10.8%) is almost double that of high school females (5.5%) and similar to cigarette use among high school males (10.6%).

## Middle School Students

Percentage of U.S. middle school students who were current cigar smokers† in 2014:

- 1.9 percent of all U.S. students in grades 6–8

- 1.4 percent of female students in grades 6–8

- 2.4 percent of male students in grades 6–8

## Overall

- In 2013, an estimated 12.4 million people in the United States aged 12 years or older (or 5.2%) were current cigar smokers.

*Adults are defined as persons 18 years of age or older.*

† *Current cigar use is defined as smoking cigars on 1 or more of the 30 days before participation in a survey about this topic.*

# Marketing Information

**Marketing efforts promote cigars as symbols of a luxury and successful lifestyle. The following strategies can contribute to the increased acceptability of cigar smoking:**

- Endorsements by celebrities

- Development of cigar-friendly magazines (e.g., Cigar Aficionado)

- Images of highly visible women smoking cigars

- Product placement in movies

In 2001, the Federal Trade Commission mandated that cigar packaging and advertisements must display one of the following five "SURGEON GENERAL WARNING" text-only labels on a rotating basis

- Cigar Smoking Can Cause Cancers Of The Mouth And Throat, Even If You Do Not Inhale.
- Cigar Smoking Can Cause Lung Cancer And Heart Disease.
- Tobacco Use Increases The Risk Of Infertility, Stillbirth, And Low Birth Weight.
- Cigars Are Not A Safe Alternative To Cigarettes.
- Tobacco Smoke Increases The Risk Of Lung Cancer And Heart Disease, Even In Nonsmokers.

# Chapter 19
# Hookah Pipes

- **Hookahs** are water pipes that are used to smoke specially made tobacco that comes in different flavors, such as apple, mint, cherry, chocolate, coconut, licorice, cappuccino, and watermelon.

  - Although many users think it is less harmful, hookah smoking has many of the same health risks as cigarette smoking.

  - Hookah is also called *narghile, argileh, shisha, hubble-bubble*, and *goza*.

  - Hookahs vary in size, shape, and style.

  - A typical modern hookah has a head (with holes in the bottom), a metal body, a water bowl, and a flexible hose with a mouthpiece.

  - Hookah smoking is typically done in groups, with the same mouthpiece passed from person to person.

---

- In 2015, more than 1 million high school students and an estimated 220,000 middle school students reported smoking hookah within the past 30 days.
- 78.9 percent of youth aged 12–17 who smoked hookah said that they used hookah products because "they come in flavors I like."

*(Source: "Hookah Tobacco (Shisha Or Waterpipe Tobacco)," U.S. Food and Drug Administration (FDA), November 7, 2016.)*

---

About This Chapter: This chapter includes text excerpted from "Hookahs," Centers for Disease Control and Prevention (CDC), February 22, 2016.

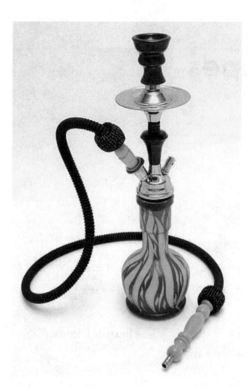

*Figure 19.1.* Hookah Pipe

# Health Effects

Using a hookah to smoke tobacco poses serious health risks to smokers and others exposed to the smoke from the hookah.

## Hookah Smoke And Cancer

- The charcoal used to heat the tobacco can raise health risks by producing high levels of carbon monoxide, metals, and cancer-causing chemicals.

- Even after it has passed through water, the smoke from a hookah has high levels of these toxic agents.

- Hookah tobacco and smoke contain several toxic agents known to cause lung, bladder, and oral cancers.

- Tobacco juices from hookahs irritate the mouth and increase the risk of developing oral cancers.

## Other Health Effects Of Hookah Smoke

- Hookah tobacco and smoke contain many toxic agents that can cause clogged arteries and heart disease.

- Infections may be passed to other smokers by sharing a hookah.

- Babies born to women who smoked water pipes every day while pregnant weigh less at birth (at least 3½ ounces less) than babies born to nonsmokers.

- Babies born to hookah smokers are also at increased risk for respiratory diseases.

## Hookah Smoking Compared With Cigarette Smoking

- While many hookah smokers may think this practice is less harmful than smoking cigarettes, hookah smoking has many of the same health risks as cigarette smoking.

  - Water pipe smoking delivers nicotine—the same highly addictive drug found in other tobacco products.

  - The tobacco in hookahs is exposed to high heat from burning charcoal, and the smoke is at least as toxic as cigarette smoke.

- Because of the way a hookah is used, smokers may absorb more of the toxic substances also found in cigarette smoke than cigarette smokers do.

  - An hour-long hookah smoking session involves 200 puffs, while smoking an average cigarette involves 20 puffs.

  - The amount of smoke inhaled during a typical hookah session is about 90,000 milliliters (ml), compared with 500–600 ml inhaled when smoking a cigarette.

- Hookah smokers may be at risk for some of the same diseases as cigarette smokers. These include:

  - Oral cancer

  - Lung cancer

  - Stomach cancer

  - Cancer of the esophagus

  - Reduced lung function

  - Decreased fertility

## Hookahs And Secondhand Smoke

Secondhand smoke from hookahs can be a health risk for nonsmokers. It contains smoke from the tobacco as well as smoke from the heat source (e.g., charcoal) used in the hookah.

## Nontobacco Hookah Products

- Some sweetened and flavored nontobacco products are sold for use in hookahs.

- Labels and ads for these products often claim that users can enjoy the same taste without the harmful effects of tobacco.

- Studies of tobacco-based shisha and "herbal" shisha show that smoke from both preparations contain carbon monoxide and other toxic agents known to increase the risks for smoking-related cancers, heart disease, and lung disease.

# Chapter 20
# Secondhand Smoke

## What Is Secondhand Smoke?

Secondhand smoke is the combination of smoke that comes from a cigarette and smoke breathed out by a smoker. When a non-smoker is around someone smoking, they breathe in secondhand smoke.

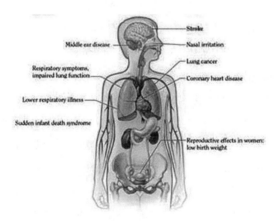

***Figure 20.1.*** Health Consequences Causally Linked To Exposure To Secondhand Smoke

*Source: "Smoking And Tobacco Use: Health Effects of Secondhand Smoke," Centers for Disease Control and Prevention (CDC), February 17, 2016.*

About This Chapter: Text beginning with the heading "What Is Secondhand Smoke?" is excerpted from "Protect Your Loved Ones From Secondhand Smoke," Smokefree.gov, U.S. Department of Health and Human Services (HHS), July 30, 2013. Reviewed December 2016; Text beginning with the heading "Patterns Of Secondhand Smoke Exposure" is excerpted from "Secondhand Smoke (SHS) Facts," Centers for Disease Control and Prevention (CDC), February 17, 2016.

# Is Secondhand Smoke Dangerous?

Secondhand smoke is dangerous to anyone who breathes it in. There is no safe amount of secondhand smoke. It contains over 7,000 harmful chemicals, at least 250 of which are known to damage your health. It can also stay in the air for several hours after somebody smokes. Even breathing secondhand smoke for a short amount of time can hurt your body.

Over time, secondhand smoke can cause serious health issues like cancer and heart disease in non-smokers. Here are a few of the ways secondhand smoke harms your body:

- **Cancer.** It has more than 70 toxic chemicals known to cause cancer. Secondhand smoke causes lung cancer in people who have never smoked themselves.

- **Heart disease.** Breathing secondhand smoke makes it more likely that you will get heart disease, have a heart attack, and die early.

- **Breathing problems.** It can cause coughing, extra phlegm, wheezing, and shortness of breath.

Secondhand smoke is especially dangerous for children, babies, and women who are pregnant. Some of the more serious health effects include:

- **SIDS (sudden infant death syndrome).** Babies whose moms smoke while pregnant or who are exposed to secondhand smoke after birth are more likely to die from SIDS.

- **Smaller babies.** Mothers who breathe secondhand smoke while pregnant are more likely to have smaller babies. Babies born small are weaker and have a higher risk for many serious health problems.

- **Weak lungs.** Babies who breathe secondhand smoke after birth have weaker lungs than other babies. This increases their risk of many health problems.

- **Severe asthma.** Secondhand smoke causes kids who already have asthma to get more frequent and severe attacks.

- **Breathing problems.** Kids whose parents smoke around them get bronchitis and pneumonia more often. Secondhand smoke also causes lung problems, including coughing, too much phlegm, wheezing, and breathlessness among school-aged kids.

- **Ear infections.** Kids exposed to secondhand smoke are more likely to get ear infections.

The only way to fully protect non-smokers from the dangers of secondhand smoke is to not allow smoking indoors. Separating smokers from nonsmokers (like "no smoking" sections in restaurants), cleaning the air, and airing out buildings does not completely get rid of secondhand smoke.

# How Can I Protect My Loved Ones From Secondhand Smoke?

The best thing you can do to protect your family from secondhand smoke is to quit smoking. Right away, you get rid of their exposure to secondhand smoke in your home and car, and reduce it anywhere else you go together.

Another important step is to make sure your house and car remain smokefree. Kids breathe in secondhand smoke at home more than any other place. The same goes for many adults. Set "smokefree rules" for anyone in your home or car. Setting these rules can:

- Reduce the amount of secondhand smoke your family breathes in
- Help you quit smoking and stay smokefree
- Lower the chance of your child becoming a smoker

Whether at home or on the go, there are steps you can take to protect your family from secondhand smoke. These include:

- Asking people not to smoke in your home or car
- Making sure people looking after your children (e.g., nannies, babysitters, day care) do not smoke
- Choosing smokefree restaurants
- Avoiding indoor public places that allow smoking
- Teaching your children to stay away from secondhand smoke

# Patterns Of Secondhand Smoke Exposure

## Secondhand Smoke Exposure Has Decreased In Recent Years

- Measurements of cotinine show that exposure to secondhand smoke has steadily decreased in the United States over time.
  - During 2011–2012, about 25 of every 100 (25.3%) nonsmokers had measurable levels of cotinine.
- The decrease in exposure to secondhand smoke is likely due to:
  - The growing number of states and communities with laws that do not allow smoking in indoor areas of workplaces and public places, including restaurants, bars, and casinos

- The growing number of households with voluntary smokefree home rules

- Significant declines in cigarette smoking rates

- The fact that smoking around nonsmokers has become much less socially acceptable

## Many People In The United States Are Still Exposed To Secondhand Smoke

- During 2011–2012, about 58 million nonsmokers in the United States were exposed to secondhand smoke.

- Among children who live in homes in which no one smokes indoors, those who live in multi-unit housing (for example, apartments or condos) have 45 percent higher cotinine levels (or almost half the amount) than children who live in single-family homes.

- During 2011–2012, 2 out of every 5 children ages 3 to 11—including 7 out of every 10 Black children—in the United States were exposed to secondhand smoke regularly.

- During 2011–2012, more than 1 in 3 (36.8%) nonsmokers who lived in rental housing were exposed to secondhand smoke.

# What You Can Do

You can protect yourself and your family from secondhand smoke by:

- Quitting smoking if you are not already a nonsmoker

- Not allowing anyone to smoke anywhere in or near your home

- Not allowing anyone to smoke in your car, even with the windows down

- Seeking out restaurants and other places that do not allow smoking (if your state still allows smoking in public areas)

- Being a good role model by not smoking or using any other type of tobacco

# Chapter 21
# Smokeless Tobacco

## What Is Smokeless Tobacco?

Smokeless tobacco:

- Is not burned

- Includes tobacco that can be sucked or chewed

- Can be spit or swallowed, depending on the product

- Can be spitless, depending on the product

- Contains nicotine and is addictive

- May appeal to youth because it comes in flavors such as cinnamon, berry, vanilla, and apple

Types of smokeless tobacco:

- Chewing tobacco (loose leaf, plug, or twist and may come in flavors)

- Snuff (moist, dry, or in packets [U.S. snus])

- Dissolvables (lozenges, sticks, strips, orbs)

### Chewing Tobacco

Chewing tobacco comes in the form of loose leaf, plug, or twist.

About This Chapter: Text under the heading "What Is Smokeless Tobacco?" is excerpted from "Smokeless Tobacco: Products And Marketing," Centers for Disease Control and Prevention (CDC), May 9, 2016; Text beginning with the heading "Smokeless Tobacco: Health Effects" is excerpted from "Smokeless Tobacco: Health Effects," Centers for Disease Control and Prevention (CDC), February 18, 2016.

**Table 21.1.** Types Of Chewing Tobacco

| Form | Description | Use | Market Share (in 2011)* |
|---|---|---|---|
| Loose leaf | Cured (aged) tobacco, typically sweetened and packaged in foil pouches | Piece taken from pouch and placed between cheek and gums | 17.50% |
| Plug | Cured tobacco leaves pressed together into a cake or "plug" form and wrapped in a tobacco leaf | Piece taken from pouch and placed between cheek and gums | 0.50% |
| Twist or roll | Cured (aged) tobacco leaves twisted together like a rope | Piece cut off from twist and placed between cheek and gums | 0.20% |

*\* Market share is the percentage of the U.S. smokeless tobacco market for a specific product. For example, almost 2 of every 10 smokeless products (17.5%) sold in the United States in 2011 were loose-leaf smokeless tobacco products.*

## Snuff

Snuff is finely ground tobacco that can be dry, moist, or packaged in pouches or packets (dip, U.S. snus).

- Some types of snuff are sniffed or inhaled into the nose; other types are placed in the mouth.

- Snus is a newer form of moist snuff used in the United States.

**Table 21.2.** Forms Of Snuff

| Form | Description | Use | Market Share (in 2011)* |
|---|---|---|---|
| Moist | Cured (aged) and fermented tobacco processed into fine particles and often packaged in round cans | Pinch or "dip" is placed between cheek or lip and gums; requires spitting | 80.70% |
| Dry | Fire-cured tobacco in powder form | Pinch of powder is put in the mouth or inhaled through the nose; may require spitting | 1.10% |

**Table 21.2.** Continued

| Form | Description | Use | Market Share (in 2011)* |
|---|---|---|---|
| U.S. snus | Moist snuff packaged in ready-to-use pouches that resemble small tea bags | Pouch is placed between cheek or teeth and gums; does not require spitting | - |

*Market share is the percentage of the U.S. smokeless tobacco market for a specific product. For example, more than 8 of every 10 snuff products sold in the United States in 2011 were moist snuff products.*

## Other Tobacco Products That Are Not Burned

Dissolvables are finely ground tobacco pressed into shapes such as tablets, sticks, or strips.

- Dissolvable tobacco products slowly dissolve in the mouth.

- These products may appeal to youth because they come in attractive packaging, look like candy or small mints, and can be easily hidden from view.

**Table 21.3.** Forms Of Other Tobacco

| Form | Description | Market Share (in 2011) |
|---|---|---|
| Lozenges | Resemble pellets or tablets | - |
| Orbs | Resemble small mints | - |
| Sticks | Have a toothpick-like appearance | - |
| Strips | Thin sheets that work like dissolvable breath strips or medication strips | - |

# Health Effects Of Smokeless Tobacco

Smokeless tobacco is associated with many health problems. Using smokeless tobacco:

- Can lead to nicotine addiction

- Causes cancer of the mouth, esophagus (the passage that connects the throat to the stomach), and pancreas (a gland that helps with digestion and maintaining proper blood sugar levels)

- Is associated with diseases of the mouth

- Can increase risks for early delivery and stillbirth when used during pregnancy

- Can cause nicotine poisoning in children
- May increase the risk for death from heart disease and stroke

## Addiction To Smokeless Tobacco

- Smokeless tobacco contains nicotine, which is highly addictive.
- Because young people who use smokeless tobacco can become addicted to nicotine, they may be more likely to also become cigarette smokers.

## Smokeless Tobacco And Cancer

- Many smokeless tobacco products contain cancer-causing chemicals.
  - The most harmful chemicals are tobacco-specific nitrosamines, which form during the growing, curing, fermenting, and aging of tobacco. The amount of these chemicals varies by product.
  - The higher the levels of these chemicals, the greater the risk for cancer.
  - Other chemicals found in tobacco can also cause cancer. These include:
  - A radioactive element (polonium-210) found in tobacco fertilizer
  - Chemicals formed when tobacco is cured with heat (polynuclear aromatic hydrocarbons—also known as polycyclic aromatic hydrocarbons)
  - Harmful metals (arsenic, beryllium, cadmium, chromium, cobalt, lead, nickel, mercury)
- Smokeless tobacco causes cancer of the mouth, esophagus, and pancreas.

## Reproductive And Developmental Risks

- Using smokeless tobacco during pregnancy can increase the risk for early delivery and stillbirth.
- Nicotine in smokeless tobacco products that are used during pregnancy can affect how a baby's brain develops before birth.

## Other Risks

- Using smokeless tobacco increases the risk for death from heart disease and stroke.

# Part Three
## Cancers Associated With Tobacco Use

# Chapter 22

# Questions And Answers About Smoking And Cancer

## What Is Cancer?

Cancer refers to diseases in which abnormal cells divide out of control and are able to invade other tissues. Cancer cells can spread to other parts of the body through the blood and lymph systems, which help the body get rid of toxins.

There are more than 100 different types of cancer. Most cancers are named for the organ or type of cell in which they start—for example, lung cancer begins in the lung and laryngeal cancer begins in the larynx (voice box).

Symptoms can include:

- A thickening or lump in any part of the body
- Weight loss or gain with no known reason
- A sore that does not heal
- Hoarseness or a cough that does not go away
- A hard time swallowing
- Discomfort after eating
- Changes in bowel or bladder habits
- Unusual bleeding or discharge
- Feeling weak or very tired

About This Chapter: Text beginning with the heading "What Is Cancer?" is excerpted from "Cancer," Centers for Disease Control and Prevention (CDC), June 22, 2016; Text beginning with the heading "Does Quitting Smoking Lower The Risk Of Cancer?" is excerpted from "Harms Of Cigarette Smoking And Health Benefits Of Quitting," National Cancer Institute (NCI), December 3, 2014.

# How Is Smoking Related To Cancer?

Smoking can cause cancer and then block your body from fighting it:

- Poisons in cigarette smoke can weaken the body's immune system, making it harder to kill cancer cells. When this happens, cancer cells keep growing without being stopped.

- Poisons in tobacco smoke can damage or change a cell's deoxyribonucleic acid (DNA). DNA is the cell's "instruction manual" that controls a cell's normal growth and function. When DNA is damaged, a cell can begin growing out of control and create a cancer tumor.

Doctors have known for years that smoking causes most lung cancers. It's still true today, when nearly 9 out of 10 lung cancers are caused by smoking cigarettes. In fact, smokers have a greater risk for lung cancer today than they did in 1964, even though they smoke fewer cigarettes. One reason may be changes in how cigarettes are made and what chemicals they contain.

Treatments are getting better for lung cancer, but it still kills more men and women than any other type of cancer. In the United States, more than 7,300 nonsmokers die each year from lung cancer caused by secondhand smoke. Secondhand smoke is the combination of smoke from the burning end of a cigarette and the smoke breathed out by smokers.

# What Are The Possible Cancers Of Smoking?

Smoking can cause cancer almost anywhere in your body, including the:

- blood (acute myeloid leukemia)
- bladder
- cervix
- colon and rectum
- esophagus
- kidneys and ureters
- larynx
- liver
- lungs
- mouth, nose, and throat

- pancreas

- stomach

- trachea

Men with prostate cancer who smoke may be more likely to die from these diseases than nonsmokers.

Smokeless tobacco, such as chewing tobacco, also causes cancer, including cancers of the:

- esophagus

- mouth and throat

- pancreas

# How Can Smoking-Related Cancers Be Prevented?

Quitting smoking lowers the risks for cancers of the lung, mouth, throat, esophagus, and larynx.

- Within 5 years of quitting, your chance of getting cancer of the mouth, throat, esophagus, and bladder is cut in half.

- Ten years after you quit smoking, your risk of dying from lung cancer drops by half.

If nobody smoked, one of every three cancer deaths in the United States would not happen.

# How Is Cancer Treated?

The treatment for cancer depends on the type of cancer and the stage of the disease (how severe the cancer is and whether it has spread). Doctors may also consider the patient's age and general health. Often, the goal of treatment is to cure the cancer. In other cases, the goal is to control the disease or to reduce symptoms for as long as possible. The treatment plan for a person may change over time.

Most treatment plans include surgery, radiation therapy, or chemotherapy. Other plans involve biological therapy (a treatment that helps your immune system fight cancer).

Some cancers respond best to a single type of treatment. Other cancers may respond best to a combination of treatments.

For patients who get very high doses of chemotherapy or radiation therapy, a stem cell transplant, also known as a bone marrow transplant, may be recommended by their doctor.

This is because high-dose therapies destroy both cancer cells and normal blood cells. A stem cell transplant can help the body to make healthy blood cells to replace the ones lost due to the cancer treatment. It's a complicated procedure with many side effects and risks.

Quitting smoking improves the outlook (the prognosis) for people with cancer. People who continue to smoke after diagnosis raise their risk for future cancers and death. They are more likely to die from cancer than nonsmokers and are more likely to develop a second (new) tobacco-related cancer.

# Does Quitting Smoking Lower The Risk Of Cancer?

Yes. Quitting smoking reduces the risk of developing and dying from cancer. Although it is never too late to get a benefit from quitting, the benefit is strongest among those who quit at a younger age.

The risk of premature death and the chance of developing cancer from smoking depend on many factors, including the number of years a person smokes, the number of cigarettes he or she smokes per day, the age at which he or she began smoking, and whether or not he or she was already ill at the time of quitting. For people who have already developed cancer, quitting smoking reduces the risk of developing a second cancer.

---

If you quit smoking right now...

- Within 20 minutes: Your heart rate and blood pressure drop.
- Within 12 hours: The carbon monoxide level in your blood drops to normal.
- Within 3 months: Your circulation and lung function improves.
- Within 9 months: You will cough less and breathe easier.
- After 1 year: Your risk of coronary heart disease is cut in half.
- After 5 years: Your risk of cancer of the mouth, throat, esophagus, and bladder are cut in half. Your risk of cervical cancer and stroke return to normal after 5 years.
- After 10 years: You are half as likely to die from lung cancer. Your risk of larynx or pancreatic cancer decreases.
- After 15 years: Your risk of coronary heart disease is the same as a non-smoker's.

*(Source: "Get On The Path To A Healthier You," BeTobaccoFree.gov, November 15, 2012.)*

---

# Should Someone Already Diagnosed With Cancer Bother To Quit Smoking?

Yes. Cigarette smoking has a profound adverse impact on health outcomes in cancer patients. For patients with some cancers, quitting smoking at the time of diagnosis may reduce the risk of dying by 30 percent to 40 percent. For those having surgery, chemotherapy, or other treatments, quitting smoking helps improve the body's ability to heal and respond to therapy. It also lowers the risk of pneumonia and respiratory failure. Moreover, quitting smoking may lower the risk of the cancer returning, of dying from the cancer, of a second cancer developing, and of dying from other causes.

# Chapter 23
# Bladder Cancer

The bladder is a hollow organ in the lower part of the abdomen. It is shaped like a small balloon and has a muscular wall that allows it to get larger or smaller to store urine made by the kidneys. There are two kidneys, one on each side of the backbone, above the waist. Tiny tubules in the kidneys filter and clean the blood. They take out waste products and make urine. The urine passes from each kidney through a long tube called a ureter into the bladder. The bladder holds the urine until it passes through the urethra and leaves the body.

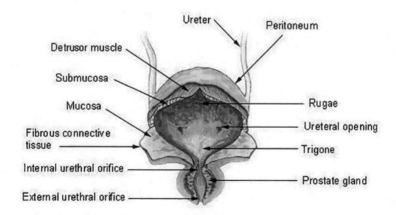

***Figure 23.1.*** Urinaray Bladder

*(Source: "Urinary Bladder," National Cancer Institute (NCI), July 1, 2002.)*

About This Chapter: This chapter includes text excerpted from "Bladder Cancer Treatment (PDQ®)—Patient Version," National Cancer Institute (NCI), July 7, 2016.

# Risk Factors

Anything that increases your chance of getting a disease is called a risk factor. Having a risk factor does not mean that you will get cancer; not having risk factors doesn't mean that you will not get cancer. Talk to your doctor if you think you may be at risk for bladder cancer.

Risk factors for bladder cancer include:

- Using tobacco, especially smoking cigarettes.

- Having a family history of bladder cancer.

- Having certain changes in the genes that are linked to bladder cancer.

- Being exposed to paints, dyes, metals, or petroleum products in the workplace.

- Past treatment with radiation therapy to the pelvis or with certain anticancer drugs, such as cyclophosphamide or ifosfamide.

- Taking *Aristolochia fangchi*, a Chinese herb.

- Drinking water from a well that has high levels of arsenic.

- Drinking water that has been treated with chlorine.

- Having a history of bladder infections, including bladder infections caused by *Schistosoma haematobium*.

- Using urinary catheters for a long time.

Older age is a risk factor for most cancers. The chance of getting cancer increases as you get older.

# Signs And Symptoms

These and other signs and symptoms may be caused by bladder cancer or by other conditions. Check with your doctor if you have any of the following:

- blood in the urine (slightly rusty to bright red in color)

- frequent urination

- lower back pain

- pain during urination

# Diagnosis Test

The following tests and procedures may be used:

- biopsy
- cystoscopy
- internal exam
- intravenous pyelogram (IVP)
- physical exam and history
- urinalysis
- urine cytology

# Prognosis And Treatment Options

The prognosis (chance of recovery) depends on the following:

- The stage of the cancer (whether it is superficial or invasive bladder cancer, and whether it has spread to other places in the body). Bladder cancer in the early stages can often be cured.
- The type of bladder cancer cells and how they look under a microscope.
- Whether there is carcinoma in situ in other parts of the bladder.
- The patient's age and general health.

If the cancer is superficial, prognosis also depends on the following:

- How many tumors there are.
- The size of the tumors.
- Whether the tumor has recurred (come back) after treatment.

Treatment options depend on the stage of bladder cancer.

# Treatment Option Overview

- There are different types of treatment for patients with bladder cancer.
- Four types of standard treatment are used:
  - Surgery

- Radiation therapy

- Chemotherapy

- Biologic therapy

- New types of treatment are being tested in clinical trials.

- Patients may want to think about taking part in a clinical trial.

- Patients can enter clinical trials before, during, or after starting their cancer treatment.

- Follow-up tests may be needed.

# Chapter 24
# Colorectal Cancer

The colon and the rectum are parts of the large intestine, which is the lower part of the body's digestive system. During digestion, food moves through the stomach and small intestine into the colon. The colon absorbs water and nutrients from the food and stores waste matter (stool). Stool moves from the colon into the rectum before it leaves the body.

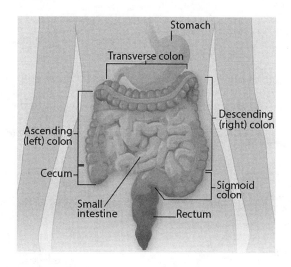

*Figure 24.1.* Colon And Rectum

*(Source: "Colorectal (Colon) Cancer," Centers for Disease Control and Prevention (CDC), April 25, 2016.)*

---

About This Chapter: This chapter includes text excerpted from "Colorectal Cancer—Patient Version," National Cancer Institute (NCI), June 30, 2016.

Most colorectal cancers are adenocarcinomas (cancers that begin in cells that make and release mucus and other fluids). Colorectal cancer often begins as a growth called a polyp, which may form on the inner wall of the colon or rectum. Some polyps become cancer over time. Finding and removing polyps can prevent colorectal cancer.

Colorectal cancer is the third most common type of cancer in men and women in the United States. Deaths from colorectal cancer have decreased with the use of colonoscopies and fecal occult blood tests, which check for blood in the stool.

# Colon Cancer Treatment

## Risk Factors

Anything that increases your chance of getting a disease is called a risk factor. Having a risk factor does not mean that you will get cancer; not having risk factors doesn't mean that you will not get cancer. Talk with your doctor if you think you may be at risk. Risk factors include the following:

- Tobacco use.

- Certain hereditary conditions, such as familial adenomatous polyposis and hereditary nonpolyposis colon cancer (HNPCC; Lynch Syndrome).

- A history of ulcerative colitis (ulcers in the lining of the large intestine) or Crohn's disease.

- A personal history of cancer of the colon, rectum, ovary, endometrium, or breast.

- A personal history of polyps (small areas of bulging tissue) in the colon or rectum.

## Signs And Symptoms

These and other signs and symptoms may be caused by colon cancer or by other conditions. Check with your doctor if you have any of the following:

- A change in bowel habits

- Blood (either bright red or very dark) in the stool.

- Diarrhea, constipation, or feeling that the bowel does not empty all the way.

- Stools that are narrower than usual

- Frequent gas pains, bloating, fullness, or cramps

- Weight loss for no known reason

- Feeling very tired

- Vomiting

## Diagnosis Test

The following tests and procedures may be used:

- barium enema

- biopsy

- colonoscopy

- digital rectal exam

- fecal occult blood test

- physical exam and history

- sigmoidoscopy

- virtual colonoscopy

## Prognosis And Treatment Options

The prognosis (chance of recovery) and treatment options depend on the following:

- The stage of the cancer (whether the cancer is in the inner lining of the colon only or has spread through the colon wall, or has spread to lymph nodes or other places in the body).

- Whether the cancer has blocked or made a hole in the colon.

- Whether there are any cancer cells left after surgery.

- Whether the cancer has recurred.

- The patient's general health.

The prognosis also depends on the blood levels of carcinoembryonic antigen (CEA) before treatment begins. CEA is a substance in the blood that may be increased when cancer is present.

## Treatment Option Overview

- There are different types of treatment for patients with colon cancer.

- Six types of standard treatment are used:
  - Chemotherapy
  - Cryosurgery
  - Radiation therapy
  - Radiofrequency ablation
  - Surgery
  - Targeted therapy
- New types of treatment are being tested in clinical trials.
- Patients may want to think about taking part in a clinical trial.
- Patients can enter clinical trials before, during, or after starting their cancer treatment.
- Follow-up tests may be needed.

# Rectal Cancer Treatment

The rectum is part of the body's digestive system. The digestive system takes in nutrients (vitamins, minerals, carbohydrates, fats, proteins, and water) from foods and helps pass waste material out of the body. The digestive system is made up of the esophagus, stomach, and the small and large intestines. The colon (large bowel) is the first part of the large intestine and is about 5 feet long. Together, the rectum and anal canal make up the last part of the large intestine and are 6-8 inches long. The anal canal ends at the anus (the opening of the large intestine to the outside of the body).

## Risk Factors

Anything that increases your chance of getting a disease is called a risk factor. Having a risk factor does not mean that you will get cancer; not having risk factors doesn't mean that you will not get cancer. Talk with your doctor if you think you may be at risk. The following are possible risk factors for rectal cancer:

- Being aged 50 or older
- Having certain hereditary conditions, such as familial adenomatous polyposis (FAP) and hereditary nonpolyposis colon cancer (HNPCC or Lynch syndrome).
- Having a personal history of any of the following:

- Colorectal cancer

- Polyps (small pieces of bulging tissue) in the colon or rectum.

- Cancer of the ovary, endometrium, or breast

- Having a parent, brother, sister, or child with a history of colorectal cancer or polyps.

## Signs And Symptoms

These and other signs and symptoms may be caused by rectal cancer or by other conditions. Check with your doctor if you have any of the following:

- Blood (either bright red or very dark) in the stool

- A change in bowel habits

- Diarrhea

- Constipation

- Feeling that the bowel does not empty completely

- Stools that are narrower or have a different shape than usual

- General abdominal discomfort (frequent gas pains, bloating, fullness, or cramps).

- Change in appetite

- Weight loss for no known reason

- Feeling very tired

## Diagnose Test

Tests used to diagnose rectal cancer include the following:

- physical exam and history

- digital rectal exam (DRE)

- colonoscopy

- biopsy

  - reverse-transcription polymerase chain reaction (RT-PCR) test

  - immunohistochemistry

- carcinoembryonic antigen (CEA) assay

## Prognosis And Treatment Options

The prognosis (chance of recovery) and treatment options depend on the following:

- The stage of the cancer (whether it affects the inner lining of the rectum only, involves the whole rectum, or has spread to lymph nodes, nearby organs, or other places in the body).

- Whether the tumor has spread into or through the bowel wall.

- Where the cancer is found in the rectum.

- Whether the bowel is blocked or has a hole in it.

- Whether all of the tumor can be removed by surgery.

- The patient's general health.

- Whether the cancer has just been diagnosed or has recurred (come back).

## Treatment Option Overview

- There are different types of treatment for patients with rectal cancer.

- Four types of standard treatment are used:

  - Surgery

  - Radiation therapy

  - Chemotherapy

  - Targeted therapy

- Other types of treatment are being tested in clinical trials.

- Patients may want to think about taking part in a clinical trial.

- Patients can enter clinical trials before, during, or after starting their cancer treatment.

- Follow-up tests may be needed.

---

Colorectal cancer is the fourth most common cancer in the United States and the second leading cause of death from cancer.

*(Source: "Colorectal Cancer Awareness Month," Healthfinder.gov, August 18, 2016.)*

---

# Chapter 25
# Cervical Cancer

The cervix is the lower, narrow end of the uterus (the hollow, pear-shaped organ where a fetus grows). The cervix leads from the uterus to the vagina (birth canal).

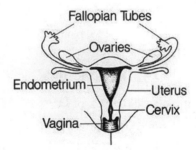

**Figure 25.1.** Cervix

*(Source: "Colorectal (Colon) Cancer," National Cancer Institute (NCI), n.d.)*

Cervical cancer usually develops slowly over time. Before cancer appears in the cervix, the cells of the cervix go through changes known as dysplasia, in which abnormal cells begin to appear in the cervical tissue. Over time, the abnormal cells may become cancer cells and start to grow and spread more deeply into the cervix and to surrounding areas.

Cervical cancer in children is rare.

---

About This Chapter: This chapter includes text excerpted from "Cervical Cancer Treatment (PDQ®)—Patient Version," National Cancer Institute (NCI), July 14, 2016.

# Risk Factors

Anything that increases your chance of getting a disease is called a risk factor. Having a risk factor does not mean that you will get cancer; not having risk factors doesn't mean that you will not get cancer. Talk to your doctor if you think you may be at risk for cervical cancer.

Risk factors for cervical cancer include the following:

- Using tobacco, especially smoking cigarettes.

- Being infected with human papillomavirus (HPV). This is the most important risk factor for cervical cancer.

- Being exposed to the drug DES (diethylstilbestrol) while in the mother's womb.

In women who are infected with HPV, the following risk factors add to the increased risk of cervical cancer:

- Giving birth to many children

- Smoking cigarettes

- Using oral contraceptives ("the Pill") for a long time

There are also risk factors that increase the risk of HPV infection:

- Having a weakened immune system caused by immunosuppression. Immunosuppression weakens the body's ability to fight infections and other diseases. The body's ability to fight HPV infection may be lowered by long-term immunosuppression from:

  - being infected with human immunodeficiency virus (HIV)

  - taking medicine to help prevent organ rejection after a transplant

- Being sexually active at a young age.

- Having many sexual partners.

Older age is a main risk factor for most cancers. The chance of getting cancer increases as you get older.

There are usually no signs or symptoms of early cervical cancer but it can be detected early with regular check-ups. Early cervical cancer may not cause signs or symptoms. Women should have regular check-ups, including tests to check for human papillomavirus (HPV) or abnormal cells in the cervix. The prognosis (chance of recovery) is better when the cancer is found early.

> ## What Is HPV?
> HPV is the most common sexually transmitted infection (STI). HPV is a different virus than HIV and HSV (herpes). HPV is so common that nearly all sexually active men and women get it at some point in their lives. There are many different types of HPV. Some types can cause health problems including genital warts and cancers.
>
> *(Source: "Genital HPV Infection—Fact Sheet," Centers for Disease Control and Prevention (CDC), April 22, 2016.)*

# Signs And Symptoms

These and other signs and symptoms may be caused by cervical cancer or by other conditions. Check with your doctor if you have any of the following:

- vaginal bleeding (including bleeding after sexual intercourse)
- unusual vaginal discharge
- pelvic pain
- pain during sexual intercourse

# Diagnosis Test

The following procedures may be used:

- biopsy
- colposcopy
- endocervical curettage
- human papillomavirus (HPV)
- pap test
- pelvic exam
- physical exam and history

# Prognosis And Treatment Options

The prognosis (chance of recovery) depends on the following:

- The stage of the cancer (the size of the tumor and whether it affects part of the cervix or the whole cervix, or has spread to the lymph nodes or other places in the body).

- The type of cervical cancer.

- The patient's age and general health.

- Whether the patient has a certain type of human papillomavirus (HPV).

- Whether the patient has human immunodeficiency virus (HIV).

- Whether the cancer has just been diagnosed or has recurred (come back).

Treatment options depend on the following:

- The stage of the cancer.

- The type of cervical cancer.

- The patient's desire to have children.

- The patient's age.

Treatment of cervical cancer during pregnancy depends on the stage of the cancer and the stage of the pregnancy. For cervical cancer found early or for cancer found during the last trimester of pregnancy, treatment may be delayed until after the baby is born.

# Treatment Option Overview

- There are different types of treatment for patients with cervical cancer.

- Four types of standard treatment are used:

  - Surgery

  - Radiation therapy

  - Chemotherapy

  - Targeted therapy

- New types of treatment are being tested in clinical trials.

- Patients may want to think about taking part in a clinical trial.

- Patients can enter clinical trials before, during, or after starting their cancer treatment.

- Follow-up tests may be needed.

# Chapter 26
# Esophageal Cancer

The esophagus is the hollow, muscular tube that moves food and liquid from the throat to the stomach. The wall of the esophagus is made up of several layers of tissue, including mucous membrane, muscle, and connective tissue.

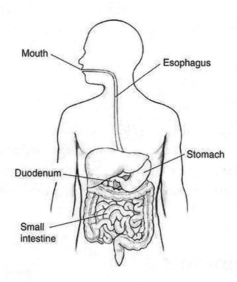

***Figure 26.1.*** Esophagus

*(Source: "Gastritis," National Institute of Diabetes and Digestive and Kidney Diseases (NIDDK), July 2015.)*

---

About This Chapter: This chapter includes text excerpted from "Esophageal Cancer Treatment (PDQ®)—Patient Version," National Cancer Institute (NCI), July 19, 2016.

Esophageal cancer starts on the inside lining of the esophagus and spreads outward through the other layers as it grows.

The two most common forms of esophageal cancer are named for the type of cells that become malignant (cancerous):

- **Squamous cell carcinoma**: Cancer that forms in squamous cells, the thin, flat cells lining the esophagus. This cancer is most often found in the upper and middle part of the esophagus, but can occur anywhere along the esophagus. This is also called epidermoid carcinoma.

- **Adenocarcinoma**: Cancer that begins in glandular (secretory) cells. Glandular cells in the lining of the esophagus produce and release fluids such as mucus. Adenocarcinomas usually form in the lower part of the esophagus, near the stomach.

# Risk Factors

Anything that increases your risk of getting a disease is called a risk factor. Having a risk factor does not mean that you will get cancer; not having risk factors doesn't mean that you will not get cancer. Talk with your doctor if you think you may be at risk. Risk factors include the following:

- Tobacco use

- Heavy alcohol use

- Barrett esophagus: A condition in which the cells lining the lower part of the esophagus have changed or been replaced with abnormal cells that could lead to cancer of the esophagus. Gastric reflux (the backing up of stomach contents into the lower section of the esophagus) may irritate the esophagus and, over time, cause Barrett esophagus.

- Older age

# Signs And Symptoms

These and other signs and symptoms may be caused by esophageal cancer or by other conditions. Check with your doctor if you have any of the following:

- painful or difficult swallowing

- weight loss

- pain behind the breastbone

- hoarseness and cough

- indigestion and heartburn

# Diagnosis Test

The following tests and procedures may be used:

- physical exam and history

- chest X-ray

- barium swallow

- esophagoscopy

- biopsy

# Prognosis And Treatment Options

The prognosis (chance of recovery) and treatment options depend on the following:

- The stage of the cancer (whether it affects part of the esophagus, involves the whole esophagus, or has spread to other places in the body).

- Whether the tumor can be completely removed by surgery.

- The patient's general health.

When esophageal cancer is found very early, there is a better chance of recovery. Esophageal cancer is often in an advanced stage when it is diagnosed. At later stages, esophageal cancer can be treated but rarely can be cured. Taking part in one of the clinical trials being done to improve treatment should be considered.

# Treatment Option Overview

- There are different types of treatment for patients with esophageal cancer.

- Patients have special nutritional needs during treatment for esophageal cancer.

- Six types of standard treatment are used:

  - surgery

  - radiation therapy

  - chemotherapy

- chemoradiation therapy

- laser therapy

- electrocoagulation

- New types of treatment are being tested in clinical trials.

    - targeted therapy

- New types of treatment are being tested in clinical trials.

- Patients may want to think about taking part in a clinical trial.

- Patients can enter clinical trials before, during, or after starting their cancer treatment.

- Follow-up tests may be needed.

---

## Esophageal cancer is found more often in men.

Men are about three times more likely than women to have esophageal cancer. There are more new cases of esophageal adenocarcinoma each year and fewer new cases of squamous cell carcinoma. Squamous cell carcinoma of the esophagus is found more often in blacks than in whites. The chance of developing esophageal cancer increases with age.

*(Source: "Esophageal Cancer Screening (PDQ®)—Patient Version," National Cancer Institute (NCI), July 27, 2015.)*

---

# Chapter 27
# Kidney Cancer

Renal cell cancer (also called kidney cancer or renal adenocarcinoma) is a disease in which malignant (cancer) cells are found in the lining of tubules (very small tubes) in the kidney. There are 2 kidneys, one on each side of the backbone, above the waist. Tiny tubules in the kidneys filter and clean the blood. They take out waste products and make urine. The urine passes from each kidney through a long tube called a ureter into the bladder. The bladder holds the urine until it passes through the urethra and leaves the body.

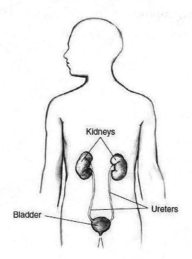

*Figure 27.1.* Kidneys

*(Source: "Ectopic Kidney," National Institute of Diabetes and Digestive and Kidney Diseases (NIDDK), June 2012.)*

About This Chapter: This chapter includes text excerpted from "Renal Cell Cancer Treatment (PDQ®)—Patient Version," National Cancer Institute (NCI), July 7, 2016.

Cancer that starts in the ureters or the renal pelvis (the part of the kidney that collects urine and drains it to the ureters) is different from renal cell cancer.

# Risk Factors

Anything that increases your risk of getting a disease is called a risk factor. Having a risk factor does not mean that you will get cancer; not having risk factors doesn't mean that you will not get cancer. Talk with your doctor if you think you may be at risk. Risk factors for renal cell cancer include the following:

- Smoking
- Misusing certain pain medicines, including over-the-counter pain medicines, for a long time.
- Having certain genetic conditions, such as von Hippel-Lindau disease or hereditary papillary renal cell carcinoma.

# Signs And Symptoms

These and other signs and symptoms may be caused by renal cell cancer or by other conditions. There may be no signs or symptoms in the early stages. Signs and symptoms may appear as the tumor grows. Check with your doctor if you have any of the following:

- blood in the urine
- a lump in the abdomen
- a pain in the side that doesn't go away
- loss of appetite
- weight loss for no known reason
- anemia

# Diagnosis Test

The following tests and procedures may be used:

- physical exam and history
- ultrasound exam
- blood chemistry studies

- urinalysis

- liver function test

- intravenous pyelogram (IVP)

- CT scan (CAT scan)

- MRI (magnetic resonance imaging)

- biopsy

# Prognosis And Treatment Options

The prognosis (chance of recovery) and treatment options depend on the following:

- The stage of the disease.

- The patient's age and general health.

# Treatment Option Overview

- There are different types of treatment for patients with renal cell cancer.

- Five types of standard treatment are used:

  - Surgery

  - Radiation therapy

  - Chemotherapy

  - Biologic therapy

  - Targeted therapy

- New types of treatment are being tested in clinical trials.

- Patients may want to think about taking part in a clinical trial.

- Patients can enter clinical trials before, during, or after starting their cancer treatment.

- Follow-up tests may be needed.

# Chapter 28

# Laryngeal Cancer

The larynx is a part of the throat, between the base of the tongue and the trachea. The larynx contains the vocal cords, which vibrate and make sound when air is directed against them. The sound echoes through the pharynx, mouth, and nose to make a person's voice.

There are three main parts of the larynx:

- **Supraglottis:** The upper part of the larynx above the vocal cords, including the epiglottis.

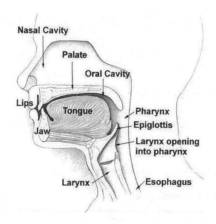

***Figure 28.1.*** *Larynx*

*(Source: "Head And Neck Overview," National Cancer Institute (NCI), September 8, 2016.)*

About This Chapter: This chapter includes text excerpted from "Laryngeal Cancer Treatment (PDQ®)—Patient Version," National Cancer Institute (NCI), May 6, 2016.

- **Glottis:** The middle part of the larynx where the vocal cords are located.

- **Subglottis:** The lower part of the larynx between the vocal cords and the trachea(windpipe).

Most laryngeal cancers form in squamous cells, the thin, flat cells lining the inside of the larynx.

Laryngeal cancer is a type of head and neck cancer.

## Risk Factors

Anything that increases your risk of getting a disease is called a risk factor. Having a risk factor does not mean that you will get cancer; not having risk factors doesn't mean that you will not get cancer. Talk with your doctor if you think you may be at risk. Possible risk factor is smoking.

## Signs And Symptoms

These and other signs and symptoms may be caused by laryngeal cancer or by other conditions. Check with your doctor if you have any of the following:

- A sore throat or cough that does not go away.

- Trouble or pain when swallowing.

- Ear pain

- A lump in the neck or throat.

- A change or hoarseness in the voice.

## Diagnosis Test

The following tests and procedures may be used:

- physical exam of the throat and neck

- biopsy

  - laryngoscopy

  - endoscopy

- CT scan (CAT scan)

- MRI (magnetic resonance imaging)

- PET scan (positron emission tomography scan)

- bone scan

- barium swallow

# Prognosis And Treatment Options

Prognosis (chance of recovery) depends on the following:

- The stage of the disease.

- The location and size of the tumor.

- The grade of the tumor.

- The patient's age, gender, and general health, including whether the patient is anemic.

Treatment options depend on the following:

- The stage of the disease.

- The location and size of the tumor.

- Keeping the patient's ability to talk, eat, and breathe as normal as possible.

- Whether the cancer has come back (recurred).

Smoking tobacco and drinking alcohol decrease the effectiveness of treatment for laryngeal cancer. Patients with laryngeal cancer who continue to smoke and drink are less likely to be cured and more likely to develop a second tumor. After treatment for laryngeal cancer, frequent and careful follow-up is important.

# Treatment Option Overview

- There are different types of treatment for patients with laryngeal cancer.

- Three types of standard treatment are used:

  - Radiation therapy

  - Surgery

  - Chemotherapy

- New types of treatment are being tested in clinical trials.

  - Chemoprevention

- Radiosensitizers

- Patients may want to think about taking part in a clinical trial.

- Patients can enter clinical trials before, during, or after starting their cancer treatment.

- Follow-up tests may be needed.

# Chapter 29
# Leukemia

Leukemia is cancer of the blood cells. Most blood cells form in the bone marrow. In leukemia, immature blood cells become cancer. These cells do not work the way they should and they crowd out the healthy blood cells in the bone marrow.

Different types of leukemia depend on the type of blood cell that becomes cancer. For example, lymphoblastic leukemia is a cancer of the lymphoblasts (white blood cells, which fight infection). White blood cells are the most common type of blood cell to become cancer. But red blood cells (cells that carry oxygen from the lungs to the rest of the body) and platelets (cells that clot the blood) may also become cancer.

Leukemia occurs most often in adults older than 55 years, but it is also the most common cancer in children younger than 15 years.

Leukemia can be either acute or chronic. Acute leukemia is a fast-growing cancer that usually gets worse quickly. Chronic leukemia is a slower-growing cancer that gets worse slowly over time. The treatment and prognosis for leukemia depend on the type of blood cell affected and whether the leukemia is acute or chronic.

> Although leukemia occurs most often in older adults, it is among the most common childhood cancers. Acute Lymphocytic Leukemia (ALL) accounts for approximately 75 percent of all childhood leukemias.
>
> *(Source: "A Snapshot Of Leukemia," National Cancer Institute (NCI), November 5, 2014.)*

---

About This Chapter: This chapter includes text excerpted from "Leukemia—Patient Version," National Cancer Institute (NCI), July 28, 2016.

# Adult Acute Myeloid Leukemia Treatment

Adult acute myeloid leukemia (AML) is a cancer of the blood and bone marrow. This type of cancer usually gets worse quickly if it is not treated. It is the most common type of acute leukemia in adults. AML is also called acute myelogenous leukemia, acute myeloblastic leukemia, acute granulocytic leukemia, and acute nonlymphocytic leukemia.

Leukemia may affect red blood cells, white blood cells, and platelets. Normally, the bone marrow makes blood stem cells (immature cells) that become mature blood cells over time. A blood stem cell may become a myeloid stem cell or a lymphoid stem cell. A lymphoid stem cell becomes a white blood cell.

A myeloid stem cell becomes one of three types of mature blood cells:

- Red blood cells that carry oxygen and other substances to all tissues of the body.

- White blood cells that fight infection and disease.

- Platelets that form blood clots to stop bleeding.

In AML, the myeloid stem cells usually become a type of immature white blood cell called myeloblasts (or myeloid blasts). The myeloblasts in AML are abnormal and do not become healthy white blood cells. Sometimes in AML, too many stem cells become abnormal red blood cells or platelets. These abnormal white blood cells, red blood cells, or platelets are also called leukemia cells or blasts. Leukemia cells can build up in the bone marrow and blood so there is less room for healthy white blood cells, red blood cells, and platelets. When this happens, infection, anemia, or easy bleeding may occur. The leukemia cells can spread outside the blood to other parts of the body, including the central nervous system(brain and spinal cord), skin, and gums.

# Subtypes Of AML

Most AML subtypes are based on how mature (developed) the cancer cells are at the time of diagnosis and how different they are from normal cells.

Acute promyelocytic leukemia (APL) is a subtype of AML that occurs when parts of two genes stick together. APL usually occurs in middle-aged adults. Signs of APL may include both bleeding and forming blood clots.

# Risk Factors

Anything that increases your risk of getting a disease is called a risk factor. Having a risk factor does not mean that you will get cancer; not having risk factors doesn't mean that you will not get cancer. Talk with your doctor if you think you may be at risk. Possible risk factors for AML include the following:

- Being male

- Smoking, especially after age 60

- Having had treatment with chemotherapy or radiation therapy in the past.

- Having had treatment for childhood acute lymphoblastic leukemia (ALL) in the past.

- Being exposed to radiation from an atomic bomb or to the chemical benzene.

- Having a history of a blood disorder such as myelodysplastic syndrome.

# Signs And Symptoms

The early signs and symptoms of AML may be like those caused by the flu or other common diseases. Check with your doctor if you have any of the following:

- fever

- shortness of breath

- easy bruising or bleeding

- petechiae (flat, pinpoint spots under the skin caused by bleeding)

- weakness or feeling tired

- weight loss or loss of appetite

# Diagnose Test

The following tests and procedures may be used:

- physical exam and history

- complete blood count (CBC)

- peripheral blood smear

- bone marrow aspiration and biopsy

- cytogenetic analysis

- immunophenotyping

- reverse transcription–polymerase chain reaction test (RT–PCR)

# Prognosis And Treatment Options

The prognosis (chance of recovery) and treatment options depend on:

- The age of the patient.

- The subtype of AML.

- Whether the patient received chemotherapy in the past to treat a different cancer.

- Whether there is a history of a blood disorder such as myelodysplastic syndrome.

- Whether the cancer has spread to the central nervous system.

- Whether the cancer has been treated before or recurred (come back).

It is important that acute leukemia be treated right away.

# Treatment Option Overview

- There are different types of treatment for patients with adult acute myeloid leukemia.

- The treatment of adult AML usually has 2 phases.

- Four types of standard treatment are used:

    - Chemotherapy

    - Radiation therapy

    - Stem cell transplant

    - Other drug therapy

- New types of treatment are being tested in clinical trials.

    - Targeted therapy

- Patients may want to think about taking part in a clinical trial.

- Patients can enter clinical trials before, during, or after starting their cancer treatment.

- Follow-up tests may be needed.

# Chapter 30
# Liver And Bile Duct Cancer

The liver has many important functions in the body. For example, it cleans toxins from the blood, makes bile that helps digest fat, makes substances that help blood clot, and makes, stores, and releases sugar for energy.

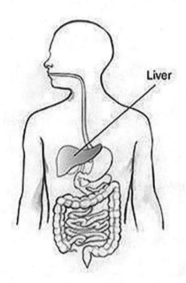

**Figure 30.1.** Liver

*(Source: "Cirrhosis," National Institute of Diabetes and Digestive and Kidney Diseases (NIDDK), November 2013.)*

About This Chapter: This chapter includes text excerpted from "Liver And Bile Duct Cancer—Patient Version," National Cancer Institute (NCI), May 15, 2015.

Primary liver cancer is cancer that starts in the liver. The most common type of primary liver cancer is hepatocellular carcinoma, which occurs in the tissue of the liver. When cancer starts in other parts of the body and spreads to the liver, it is called liver metastasis.

There are two types of liver cancer that can form in children. Hepatoblastoma occurs in younger children, and hepatocellular carcinoma occurs in older children and teenagers.

The bile ducts are tubes that carry bile between the liver and gallbladder and the intestine. Bile duct cancer is also called cholangiocarcinoma. When it begins in the bile ducts inside the liver, it is called intrahepatic cholangiocarcinoma. When it begins in the bile ducts outside the liver, it is called extrahepatic cholangiocarcinoma. Extrahepatic cholangiocarcinoma is much more common than intrahepatic cholangiocarcinoma.

# Adult Primary Liver Cancer Treatment

Adult primary liver cancer is a disease in which malignant (cancer) cells form in the tissues of the liver. The liver is one of the largest organs in the body. It has four lobes and fills the upper right side of the abdomen inside the rib cage. Three of the many important functions of the liver are:

- To filter harmful substances from the blood so they can be passed from the body in stools and urine.

- To make bile to help digest fat that comes from food.

- To store glycogen (sugar), which the body uses for energy.

## Types Of Adult Primary Liver Cancer

The two types of adult primary liver cancer are:

- Hepatocellular carcinoma.

- Cholangiocarcinoma (bile duct cancer).

The most common type of adult primary liver cancer is hepatocellular carcinoma. This type of liver cancer is the third leading cause of cancer-related deaths worldwide.

This chapter is about the treatment of primary liver cancer (cancer that begins in the liver). Treatment of cancer that begins in other parts of the body and spreads to the liver is not covered in this chapter.

Primary liver cancer can occur in both adults and children. However, treatment for children is different than treatment for adults.

## Risk Factors

Anything that increases your chance of getting a disease is called a risk factor. Having a risk factor does not mean that you will get cancer; not having risk factors doesn't mean that you will not get cancer. Talk with your doctor if you think you may be at risk.

The following are risk factors for adult primary liver cancer:

- Having hepatitis B or hepatitis C. Having both hepatitis B and hepatitis C increases the risk even more.

- Having cirrhosis, which can be caused by:

  - hepatitis (especially hepatitis C); or

  - drinking large amounts of alcohol for many years or being an alcoholic.

- Having metabolic syndrome, a set of conditions that occur together, including extra fat around the abdomen, high blood sugar, high blood pressure, high levels of triglycerides and low levels of high-density lipoproteins in the blood.

- Having liver injury that is long-lasting, especially if it leads to cirrhosis.

- Having hemochromatosis, a condition in which the body takes up and stores more iron than it needs. The extra iron is stored in the liver, heart, and pancreas

- Eating foods tainted with aflatoxin (poison from a fungus that can grow on foods, such as grains and nuts, that have not been stored properly).

- Using tobacco.

## Signs And Symptoms

These and other signs and symptoms may be caused by adult primary liver cancer or by other conditions. Check with your doctor if you have any of the following:

- A hard lump on the right side just below the rib cage.

- Discomfort in the upper abdomen on the right side.

- A swollen abdomen.

- Pain near the right shoulder blade or in the back.

- Jaundice (yellowing of the skin and whites of the eyes).

- Easy bruising or bleeding.

- Unusual tiredness or weakness.

- Nausea and vomiting

- Loss of appetite or feelings of fullness after eating a small meal.

- Weight loss for no known reason.

- Pale, chalky bowel movements and dark urine.

- Fever

## Diagnosis Test

The following tests and procedures may be used:

- physical exam and history

- serum tumor marker test

- liver function tests

- CT scan (CAT scan)

- MRI (magnetic resonance imaging)

- ultrasound exam

- biopsy

  - fine-needle aspiration biopsy

  - core needle biopsy

  - laparoscopy

## Prognosis And Treatment Options

The prognosis (chance of recovery) and treatment options depend on the following:

- The stage of the cancer (the size of the tumor, whether it affects part or all of the liver, or has spread to other places in the body).

- How well the liver is working.

- The patient's general health, including whether there is cirrhosis of the liver.

## Treatment Option Overview

- There are different types of treatment for patients with adult primary liver cancer.

- Patients with liver cancer are treated by a team of specialists who are experts in treating liver cancer.
- Seven types of standard treatment are used:
  - Surveillance
  - Surgery
  - Liver transplant
  - Ablation therapy
  - Embolization therapy
  - Targeted therapy
  - Radiation therapy
- New types of treatment are being tested in clinical trials.
- Patients may want to think about taking part in a clinical trial.
- Patients can enter clinical trials before, during, or after starting their cancer treatment.
- Follow-up tests may be needed.

# Bile Duct Cancer Treatment

Bile duct cancer is a rare disease in which malignant (cancer) cells form in the bile ducts.

A network of tubes, called ducts, connects the liver, gallbladder, and small intestine. This network begins in the liver where many small ducts collect bile (a fluid made by the liver to break down fats during digestion). The small ducts come together to form the right and left hepatic ducts, which lead out of the liver. The two ducts join outside the liver and form the common hepatic duct. The cystic duct connects the gallbladder to the common hepatic duct. Bile from the liver passes through the hepatic ducts, common hepatic duct, and cystic duct and is stored in the gallbladder.

When food is being digested, bile stored in the gallbladder is released and passes through the cystic duct to the common bile duct and into the small intestine.

Bile duct cancer is also called cholangiocarcinoma.

There are two types of bile duct cancer:

- **Intrahepatic bile duct cancer:** This type of cancer forms in the bile ducts inside the liver. Only a small number of bile duct cancers are intrahepatic. Intrahepatic bile duct cancers are also called intrahepatic cholangiocarcinomas.

- **Extrahepatic bile duct cancer:** The extrahepatic bile duct is made up of the hilum region and the distal region. Cancer can form in either region:

  - **Perihilar bile duct cancer:** This type of cancer is found in the hilum region, the area where the right and left bile ducts exit the liver and join to form the common hepatic duct. Perihilar bile duct cancer is also called a Klatskin tumor or perihilar cholangiocarcinoma.

  - **Distal extrahepatic bile duct cancer:** This type of cancer is found in the distal region. The distal region is made up of the common bile duct which passes through the pancreas and ends in the small intestine. Distal extrahepatic bile duct cancer is also called extrahepatic cholangiocarcinoma.

## Risk Factors

Anything that increases your risk of getting a disease is called a risk factor. Having a risk factor does not mean that you will get cancer; not having risk factors doesn't mean that you will not get cancer. People who think they may be at risk should discuss this with their doctor.

Risk factors for bile duct cancer include the following conditions:

- Primary sclerosing cholangitis (a progressive disease in which the bile ducts become blocked by inflammation and scarring).
- Chronic ulcerative colitis.
- Cysts in the bile ducts (cysts block the flow of bile and can cause swollen bile ducts, inflammation, and infection).
- Infection with a Chinese liver fluke parasite.
- Using tobacco.

## Signs And Symptoms

These and other signs and symptoms may be caused by bile duct cancer or by other conditions. Check with your doctor if you have any of the following:

- jaundice (yellowing of the skin or whites of the eyes)
- dark urine
- clay colored stool
- pain in the abdomen
- fever

- itchy skin

- nausea and vomiting

- weight loss for an unknown reason

## Diagnosis Test

Procedures that make pictures of the bile ducts and the nearby area help diagnose bile duct cancer and show how far the cancer has spread. The process used to find out if cancer cells have spread within and around the bile ducts or to distant parts of the body is called staging.

In order to plan treatment, it is important to know if the bile duct cancer can be removed by surgery. Tests and procedures to detect, diagnose, and stage bile duct cancer are usually done at the same time.

The following tests and procedures may be used:

- physical exam and history

- liver function tests

- carcinoembryonic antigen (CEA) and CA 19-9 tumor marker test

- CT scan (CAT scan)

- MRI (magnetic resonance imaging)

- MRCP (magnetic resonance cholangiopancreatography)

### Different procedures may be used to obtain a sample of tissue and diagnose bile duct cancer

Cells and tissues are removed during a biopsy so they can be viewed under a microscope by a pathologist to check for signs of cancer. Different procedures may be used to obtain the sample of cells and tissue. The type of procedure used depends on whether the patient is well enough to have surgery.

Types of biopsy procedures include the following:

- **Laparoscopy:** A surgical procedure to look at the organs inside the abdomen, such as the bile ducts and liver, to check for signs of cancer. Small incisions (cuts) are made in the wall of the abdomen and a laparoscope (a thin, lighted tube) is inserted into one of the incisions. Other instruments may be inserted through the same or other incisions to perform procedures such as taking tissue samples to be checked for signs of cancer.

147

- **Percutaneous transhepatic cholangiography (PTC):** A procedure used to X-ray the liver and bile ducts. A thin needle is inserted through the skin below the ribs and into the liver. Dye is injected into the liver or bile ducts and an X-ray is taken. A sample of tissue is removed and checked for signs of cancer. If the bile duct is blocked, a thin, flexible tube called a stent may be left in the liver to drain bile into the small intestine or a collection bag outside the body. This procedure may be used when a patient cannot have surgery.

- **Endoscopic retrograde cholangiopancreatography (ERCP):** A procedure used to X-ray the ducts (tubes) that carry bile from the liver to the gallbladder and from the gallbladder to the small intestine. Sometimes bile duct cancer causes these ducts to narrow and block or slow the flow of bile, causing jaundice. An endoscope is passed through the mouth and stomach and into the small intestine. Dye is injected through the endoscope (thin, tube-like instrument with a light and a lens for viewing) into the bile ducts and an X-ray is taken. A sample of tissue is removed and checked for signs of cancer. If the bile duct is blocked, a thin tube may be inserted into the duct to unblock it. This tube (or stent) may be left in place to keep the duct open. This procedure may be used when a patient cannot have surgery.

## Prognosis And Treatment Options

The prognosis (chance of recovery) and treatment options depend on the following:

- Whether the cancer is in the upper or lower part of the bile duct system.

- The stage of the cancer (whether it affects only the bile ducts or has spread to the liver, lymph nodes, or other places in the body).

- Whether the cancer has spread to nearby nerves or veins.

- Whether the cancer can be completely removed by surgery.

- Whether the patient has other conditions, such as primary sclerosing cholangitis.

- Whether the level of CA 19-9 is higher than normal.

- Whether the cancer has just been diagnosed or has recurred (come back).

Treatment options may also depend on the symptoms caused by the cancer. Bile duct cancer is usually found after it has spread and can rarely be completely removed by surgery. Palliative therapy may relieve symptoms and improve the patient's quality of life.

## Treatment Option Overview

- There are different types of treatment for patients with bile duct cancer.

- Three types of standard treatment are used:

  - Surgery

  - Radiation therapy

  - Chemotherapy

- New types of treatment are being tested in clinical trials.

  - Liver transplant

- Patients may want to think about taking part in a clinical trial.

- Patients can enter clinical trials before, during, or after starting their cancer treatment.

- Follow-up tests may be needed.

# Chapter 31

# Lung Cancer

Your lungs are organs in your chest that allow your body to take in oxygen from the air. They also help remove carbon dioxide (a waste gas that can be toxic) from your body.

The lungs' intake of oxygen and removal of carbon dioxide is called gas exchange. Gas exchange is part of breathing. Breathing is a vital function of life; it helps your body work properly.

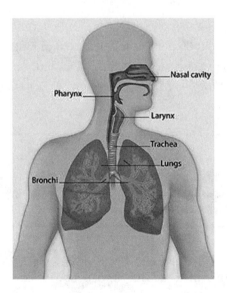

*Figure 31.1.* Lungs

About This Chapter: Text in this chapter begins with excerpts from "How The Lungs Work," National Heart, Lung, and Blood Institute (NHLBI), July 17, 2012. Reviewed December 2016; Text beginning with the heading "What Is Lung Cancer?" is excerpted from "Lung Cancer," Centers for Disease Control and Prevention (CDC), August 28, 2014.

# What Is Lung Cancer?

*Cancer* is a disease in which cells in the body grow out of control. When cancer starts in the lungs, it is called *lung cancer*.

Lung cancer begins in the lungs and may spread to lymph nodes or other organs in the body, such as the brain. Cancer from other organs also may spread to the lungs. When cancer cells spread from one organ to another, they are called *metastases*.

Lung cancers usually are grouped into two main types called small cell and non-small cell. These types of lung cancer grow differently and are treated differently. Non-small cell lung cancer is more common than small cell lung cancer.

# What Are The Risk Factors For Lung Cancer?

Research has found several risk factors that may increase your chances of getting lung cancer.

## Smoking

Cigarette smoking is the number one risk factor for lung cancer. In the United States, cigarette smoking is linked to about 80 percent to 90 percent of lung cancers. Using other tobacco products such as cigars or pipes also increases the risk for lung cancer. Tobacco smoke is a toxic mix of more than 7,000 chemicals. Many are poisons. At least 70 are known to cause cancer in people or animals.

> People who smoke cigarettes are 15 to 30 times more likely to get lung cancer or die from lung cancer than people who do not smoke. Even smoking a few cigarettes a day or smoking occasionally increases the risk of lung cancer. The more years a person smokes and the more cigarettes smoked each day, the more risk goes up.

People who quit smoking have a lower risk of lung cancer than if they had continued to smoke, but their risk is higher than the risk for people who never smoked. Quitting smoking at any age can lower the risk of lung cancer.

Cigarette smoking can cause cancer almost anywhere in the body. Cigarette smoking causes cancer of the mouth and throat, esophagus, stomach, colon, rectum, liver, pancreas, voicebox (larynx), trachea, bronchus, kidney and renal pelvis, urinary bladder, and cervix, and causes acute myeloid leukemia.

## Secondhand Smoke

Smoke from other people's cigarettes, pipes, or cigars (secondhand smoke) also causes lung cancer. When a person breathes in secondhand smoke, it is like he or she is smoking. In the United States, two out of five adults who don't smoke and half of children are exposed to secondhand smoke, and about 7,300 people who never smoked die from lung cancer due to secondhand smoke every year.

## Radon

Radon is a naturally occurring gas that comes from rocks and dirt and can get trapped in houses and buildings. It cannot be seen, tasted, or smelled. According to the U.S. Environmental Protection Agency (EPA), radon causes about 20,000 cases of lung cancer each year, making it the second leading cause of lung cancer. Nearly one out of every 15 homes in the United States is thought to have high radon levels. The EPA recommends testing homes for radon and using proven ways to lower high radon levels.

## Other Substances

Examples of substances found at some workplaces that increase risk include asbestos, arsenic, diesel exhaust, and some forms of silica and chromium. For many of these substances, the risk of getting lung cancer is even higher for those who smoke.

## Personal Or Family History Of Lung Cancer

If you are a lung cancer survivor, there is a risk that you may develop another lung cancer, especially if you smoke. Your risk of lung cancer may be higher if your parents, brothers or sisters, or children have had lung cancer. This could be true because they also smoke, or they live or work in the same place where they are exposed to radon and other substances that can cause lung cancer.

## Radiation Therapy To The Chest

Cancer survivors who had radiation therapy to the chest are at higher risk of lung cancer.

## Diet

Scientists are studying many different foods and dietary supplements to see whether they change the risk of getting lung cancer. There is much we still need to know. We do know that smokers who take beta-carotene supplements have increased risk of lung cancer.

> Many hookah smokers believe that smoking a hookah carries less risk of tobacco-related disease than cigarette smoking. However, hookah smoke contains many of the same harmful toxins as cigarette smoke and has been associated with lung cancer, respiratory illness, low birth weight, and periodontal disease.
>
> *(Source: "Dangers Of Hookah Smoking," Centers for Disease Control and Prevention (CDC), November 9, 2015.)*

# What Are The Symptoms Of Lung Cancer?

Different people have different symptoms for lung cancer. Some people have symptoms related to the lungs. Some people whose lung cancer has spread to other parts of the body (metastasized) have symptoms specific to that part of the body. Some people just have general symptoms of not feeling well. Most people with lung cancer don't have symptoms until the cancer is advanced. Lung cancer symptoms may include—

- coughing that gets worse or doesn't go away

- chest pain

- shortness of breath

- wheezing

- coughing up blood

- feeling very tired all the time

- weight loss with no known cause

Other changes that can sometimes occur with lung cancer may include repeated bouts of pneumonia and swollen or enlarged lymph nodes (glands) inside the chest in the area between the lungs.

These symptoms can happen with other illnesses, too. If you have some of these symptoms, talk to your doctor, who can help find the cause.

# What Can I Do To Reduce My Risk Of Lung Cancer?

You can help lower your risk of lung cancer in the following ways—

- **Don't smoke.** Cigarette smoking causes about 90 percent of lung cancer deaths in the United States. The most important thing you can do to prevent lung cancer is to not start smoking, or to quit if you smoke.

- **Avoid secondhand smoke.** Smoke from other people's cigarettes, cigars, or pipes is called secondhand smoke. Make your home and car smokefree.

- **Get your home tested for radon.** The U.S. Environmental Protection Agency (EPA) recommends that all homes be tested for radon.

- **Be careful at work.** Health and safety guidelines in the workplace can help workers avoid *carcinogens*—things that can cause cancer.

# What Screening Tests Are There?

Screening means testing for a disease when there are no symptoms or history of that disease. Doctors recommend a screening test to find a disease early, when treatment may work better.

The only recommended screening test for lung cancer is *low-dose computed tomography* (also called a low-dose CT scan, or LDCT). In this test, an X-ray machine scans the body and uses low doses of radiation to make detailed pictures of the lungs.

## Who Should Be Screened?

The U.S. Preventive Services Task Force (USPSTF) recommends yearly lung cancer screening with LDCT for people who—

- Have a history of heavy smoking, and

- Smoke now or have quit within the past 15 years, and

- Are between 55 and 80 years old.

*Heavy smoking* means a smoking history of 30 pack years or more. A *pack year* is smoking an average of one pack of cigarettes per day for one year. For example, a person could have a 30 pack-year history by smoking one pack a day for 30 years or two packs a day for 15 years.

## Risks Of Screening

Lung cancer screening has at least three risks—

- A lung cancer screening test can suggest that a person has lung cancer when no cancer is present. This is called a *false-positive result*. False-positive results can lead to follow-up tests and surgeries that are not needed and may have more risks.

- A lung cancer screening test can find cases of cancer that may never have caused a problem for the patient. This is called *overdiagnosis*. Overdiagnosis can lead to treatment that is not needed.

- Radiation from repeated LDCT tests can cause cancer in otherwise healthy people.

That is why lung cancer screening is recommended only for adults who have no symptoms but who are at high risk for developing the disease because of their smoking history and age.

If you are thinking about getting screened, talk to your doctor. If lung cancer screening is right for you, your doctor can refer you to a high-quality treatment facility.

The best way to reduce your risk of lung cancer is to not smoke and to avoid secondhand smoke. Lung cancer screening is not a substitute for quitting smoking.

## When Should Screening Stop?

The Task Force recommends that yearly lung cancer screening stop when the person being screened—

- Turns 81 years old, or

- Has not smoked in 15 years, or

- Develops a health problem that makes him or her unwilling or unable to have surgery if lung cancer is found.

# How Is Lung Cancer Diagnosed And Treated?

## Types Of Lung Cancer

There two main types of lung cancer are small cell lung cancer and non-small cell lung cancer. These categories refer to what the cancer cells look like under a microscope. Non-small cell lung cancer is more common than small cell lung cancer.

## Staging

If lung cancer is diagnosed, other tests are done to find out how far it has spread through the lungs, lymph nodes, and the rest of the body. This process is called *staging*. The type and stage of lung cancer tells doctors what kind of treatment you need.

## Types Of Treatment

Lung cancer is treated in several ways, depending on the type of lung cancer and how far it has spread. People with non-small cell lung cancer can be treated with surgery, chemotherapy, radiation therapy, targeted therapy, or a combination of these treatments. People with small cell lung cancer are usually treated with radiation therapy and chemotherapy.

- **Surgery.** An operation where doctors cut out cancer tissue.

- **Chemotherapy.** Using special medicines to shrink or kill the cancer. The drugs can be pills you take or medicines given in your veins, or sometimes both.

- **Radiation therapy.** Using high-energy rays (similar to X-rays) to kill the cancer.

- **Targeted therapy.** Using drugs to block the growth and spread of cancer cells. The drugs can be pills you take or medicines given in your veins.

Doctors from different specialties often work together to treat lung cancer. *Pulmonologists* are doctors who are experts in diseases of the lungs. *Surgeons* are doctors who perform operations. *Thoracic surgeons* specialize in chest, heart, and lung surgery. *Medical oncologists* are doctors who treat cancer with medicines. *Radiation oncologists* are doctors who treat cancers with radiation.

## Complementary And Alternative Medicine

Complementary and alternative medicine are medicines and health practices that are not standard cancer treatments. Complementary medicine is used in *addition* to standard treatments, and alternative medicine is used *instead of* standard treatments. Meditation, yoga, and supplements like vitamins and herbs are some examples.

Many kinds of complementary and alternative medicine have not been tested scientifically and may not be safe. Talk to your doctor about the risks and benefits before you start any kind of complementary or alternative medicine.

## Which Treatment Is Right For Me?

Choosing the treatment that is right for you may be hard. Talk to your cancer doctor about the treatment options available for your type and stage of cancer. Your doctor can explain the risks and benefits of each treatment and their side effects. *Side effects* are how your body reacts to drugs or other treatments.

Sometimes people get an opinion from more than one cancer doctor. This is called a "second opinion." Getting a second opinion may help you choose the treatment that is right for you.

# Chapter 32
# Oral Cancer

The word *oral*, both in its Latin root and in common usage, refers to the mouth. The mouth includes not only the teeth and the gums (gingiva) and their supporting connective tissues, ligaments, and bone, but also the hard and soft palate, the soft mucosal tissue lining of the mouth and throat, the tongue, the lips, the salivary glands, the chewing muscles, and the upper and lower jaws, which are connected to the skull by the temporomandibular joints.

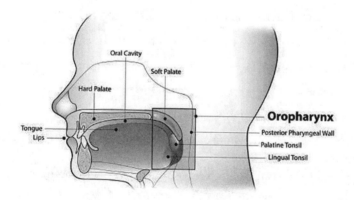

***Figure 32.1.*** Oropharynx

*(Source: "HPV And Cancer," Centers for Disease Control and Prevention (CDC), July 5, 2013.)*

About This Chapter: Text in this chapter begins with excerpts from "Chapter 1: The Meaning Of Oral Health," National Institute of Dental and Craniofacial Research (NIDCR), March 7, 2014; Text beginning with the heading "About Oral Cancer" is excerpted from "Oral Cancer," National Institute of Dental and Craniofacial Research (NIDCR), September 2016; Text under the heading "The Oral Cancer Exam" is excerpted from "The Oral Cancer Exam," National Institute of Dental and Craniofacial Research (NIDCR), August 2015.

# About Oral Cancer

- Oral cancer includes cancers of the mouth and pharynx (the back of the throat).

- Oral cancer accounts for roughly three percent of all cancers diagnosed annually in the United States. Approximately 48,000 people will be diagnosed with oral cancer each year and about 9,600 will die from the disease.

- On average, 64 percent of those with the disease will survive more than 5 years.

- Oral cancer most often occurs in people over the age of 40 and affects more than twice as many men as women.

# What Puts Someone At Risk?

**Tobacco and alcohol use.** Tobacco use of any kind, including cigarette smoking, puts you at risk. Heavy alcohol use also increases your chances of developing the disease. And using tobacco plus alcohol poses a much greater risk than using either substance alone.

**HPV.** Infection with the sexually transmitted human papillomavirus (specifically the HPV 16 type) has been linked to a subset of oral cancers.

**Age.** Risk increases with age. Oral cancer most often occurs in people over the age of 40.

**Sun Exposure.** Cancer of the lip can be caused by sun exposure.

**Diet.** A diet low in fruits and vegetables may play a role in oral cancer development.

---

## Smokeless Tobacco And Oral Disease

- Smokeless tobacco can cause white or gray patches inside the mouth (leukoplakia) that can lead to cancer.
- Smokeless tobacco can cause gum disease, tooth decay, and tooth loss.

*(Source: "Smokeless Tobacco: Health Effects," Centers for Disease Control and Prevention (CDC), December 1, 2016.)*

---

# Possible Signs And Symptoms

See a dentist or physician if any of the following symptoms lasts for more than 2 weeks.

- A sore, irritation, lump or thick patch in your mouth, lip, or throat

- A white or red patch in your mouth

- A feeling that something is caught in your throat

- Difficulty chewing or swallowing

- Difficulty moving your jaw or tongue

- Numbness in your tongue or other areas of your mouth

- Swelling of your jaw that causes dentures to fit poorly or become uncomfortable

- Pain in one ear without hearing loss

## Early Detection

It is important to find oral cancer as early as possible when it can be treated more successfully.

An oral cancer examination can detect early signs of cancer. The exam is painless and takes only a few minutes.

Your regular dental check-up is an excellent opportunity to have the exam. During the exam, your dentist or dental hygienist will check your face, neck, lips, and entire mouth for possible signs of cancer.

Some parts of the pharynx are not visible during an oral cancer exam. Talk to your dentist about whether a specialist should check your pharynx.

## The Oral Cancer Exam

An oral cancer exam is painless and quick—it takes only a few minutes. Your regular dental checkup is an excellent opportunity to have the exam.

Here's what to expect:

1. Preparing for the exam: If you have dentures (plates) or partials, you will be asked to remove them.

2. Your health care provider will inspect your face, neck, lips and mouth to look for any signs of cancer.

3. With both hands, he or she will feel the area under your jaw and the side of your neck, checking for lumps that may suggest cancer.

4. He or she will then look at and feel the insides of your lips and cheeks to check for possible signs of cancer, such as red and/or white patches.

5. Next, your provider will have you stick out your tongue so it can be checked for swelling or abnormal color or texture.

6. Using gauze, he or she will then gently pull your tongue to one side, then the other, to check the base of your tongue. The underside of your tongue will also be checked.

7. In addition, he or she will look at the roof and floor of your mouth, as well as the back of your throat.

8. Finally, your provider will put one finger on the floor of your mouth and, with the other hand under your chin, gently press down to check for lumps or sensitivity.

# Chapter 33
# Pancreatic Cancer

The pancreas is a gland about 6 inches long that is shaped like a thin pear lying on its side. The wider end of the pancreas is called the head, the middle section is called the body, and the narrow end is called the tail. The pancreas lies between the stomach and the spine.

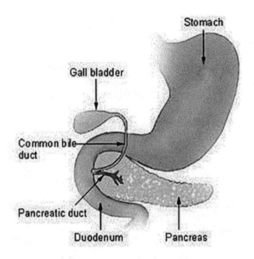

***Figure 33.1.*** Pancreas

(Source: "Pancreas," Surveillance, Epidemiology and End Results Program (SEER), National Cancer Institute (NCI), July 1, 2002.)

About This Chapter: This chapter includes text excerpted from "Pancreatic Cancer Treatment (PDQ®)—Patient Version," National Cancer Institute (NCI), June 30, 2016.

The pancreas has two main jobs in the body:

- To make juices that help digest (break down) food.

- To make hormones, such as insulin and glucagon, that help control blood sugar levels. Both of these hormones help the body use and store the energy it gets from food.

The digestive juices are made by exocrine pancreas cells and the hormones are made by endocrine pancreas cells.

About 95 percent of pancreatic cancers begin in exocrine cells.

# Risk Factors

Anything that increases your risk of getting a disease is called a risk factor. Having a risk factor does not mean that you will get cancer; not having risk factors doesn't mean that you will not get cancer. Talk with your doctor if you think you may be at risk.

Risk factors for pancreatic cancer include the following:

- Smoking

- Being very overweight

- Having a personal history of diabetes or chronic pancreatitis

- Having a family history of pancreatic cancer or pancreatitis

- Having certain hereditary conditions, such as:

  - Multiple endocrine neoplasia type 1 (MEN1) syndrome

  - Hereditary nonpolyposis colon cancer (HNPCC; Lynch syndrome)

  - von Hippel-Lindau syndrome

  - Peutz-Jeghers syndrome

  - Hereditary breast and ovarian cancer syndrome

  - Familial atypical multiple mole melanoma (FAMMM) syndrome

# Signs And Symptoms

Pancreatic cancer may not cause early signs or symptoms. Signs and symptoms may be caused by pancreatic cancer or by other conditions. Check with your doctor if you have any of the following:

- jaundice (yellowing of the skin and whites of the eyes)

- light-colored stools

- dark urine

- pain in the upper or middle abdomen and back

- weight loss for no known reason

- loss of appetite

- feeling very tired

# Diagnosis Test

Pancreatic cancer is difficult to detect and diagnose for the following reasons:

- There aren't any noticeable signs or symptoms in the early stages of pancreatic cancer.

- The signs and symptoms of pancreatic cancer, when present, are like the signs and symptoms of many other illnesses.

- The pancreas is hidden behind other organs such as the stomach, small intestine, liver, gallbladder, spleen, and bile ducts.

## Tests that examine the pancreas are used to detect, diagnose, and stage pancreatic cancer

- physical exam and history

- blood chemistry studies

- tumor marker test

- MRI (magnetic resonance imaging)

- CT scan (CAT scan)

- PET scan (positron emission tomography scan)

- abdominal ultrasound

- endoscopic ultrasound (EUS)

- endoscopic retrograde cholangiopancreatography (ERCP)

- percutaneous transhepatic cholangiography (PTC)

- laparoscopy

- biopsy

# Prognosis And Treatment Options

The prognosis (chance of recovery) and treatment options depend on the following:

- Whether or not the tumor can be removed by surgery.

- The stage of the cancer (the size of the tumor and whether the cancer has spread outside the pancreas to nearby tissues or lymph nodes or to other places in the body).

- The patient's general health.

- Whether the cancer has just been diagnosed or has recurred (come back).

Pancreatic cancer can be controlled only if it is found before it has spread, when it can be completely removed by surgery. If the cancer has spread, palliative treatment can improve the patient's quality of life by controlling the symptoms and complications of this disease.

# Treatment Option Overview

- There are different types of treatment for patients with pancreatic cancer.

- Five types of standard treatment are used:

  - Surgery

  - Radiation therapy

  - Chemotherapy

  - Chemoradiation therapy

  - Targeted therapy

- There are treatments for pain caused by pancreatic cancer.

- Patients with pancreatic cancer have special nutritional needs.

- New types of treatment are being tested in clinical trials.

  - Biologic therapy

- Patients may want to think about taking part in a clinical trial.

- Patients can enter clinical trials before, during, or after starting their cancer treatment.

- Follow-up tests may be needed

Pancreatic cancer is the 12th most common cancer in the United States, and is relatively rare; however, it is the fourth leading cause of cancer-related death in both men and women in the United States.

Cigarette smoking is the most important risk factor for pancreatic cancer.

*(Source: "A Snapshot Of Pancreatic Cancer," National Cancer Institute (NCI), November 5, 2014.)*

# Chapter 34
# Stomach Cancer

The stomach is a J-shaped organ in the upper abdomen. It is part of the digestive system, which processes nutrients (vitamins, minerals, carbohydrates, fats, proteins, and water) in foods that are eaten and helps pass waste material out of the body. Food moves from the throat to the stomach through a hollow, muscular tube called the esophagus. After leaving the stomach, partly-digested food passes into the small intestine and then into the large intestine.

The wall of the stomach is made up of 3 layers of tissue: the mucosal (innermost) layer, the muscularis (middle) layer, and the serosal (outermost) layer.

Gastric cancer begins in the cells lining the mucosal layer and spreads through the outer layers as it grows.

Stromal tumors of the stomach begin in supporting connective tissue and are treated differently from gastric cancer.

## Risk Factors

Anything that increases your risk of getting a disease is called a risk factor. Having a risk factor does not mean that you will get cancer; not having risk factors doesn't mean that you will not get cancer. Talk with your doctor if you think you may be at risk. Risk factors for gastric cancer include the following:

- Having any of the following medical conditions:

  - Helicobacter pylori (H. pylori) infection of the stomach.

About This Chapter: This chapter includes text excerpted from "Gastric Cancer Treatment (PDQ®)—Patient Version," National Cancer Institute (NCI), July 1, 2016.

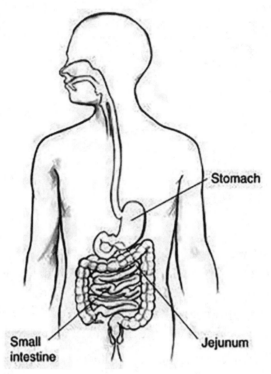

**Figure 34.1.** Stomach

*(Source: "Gastroparesis," National Institute of Diabetes and Digestive and Kidney Diseases (NIDDK), June 2012.)*

- Chronic gastritis (inflammation of the stomach)

- Pernicious anemia

- Intestinal metaplasia (a condition in which the normal stomach lining is replaced with the cells that line the intestines)

- Familial adenomatous polyposis (FAP) or gastric polyps.

- Eating a diet high in salted, smoked foods and low in fruits and vegetables.

- Eating foods that have not been prepared or stored properly.

- Being older or male.

- Smoking cigarettes

- Having a mother, father, sister, or brother who has had stomach cancer.

# Signs And Symptoms

These and other signs and symptoms may be caused by gastric cancer or by other conditions.

In the early stages of gastric cancer, the following symptoms may occur:

- indigestion and stomach discomfort
- a bloated feeling after eating
- mild nausea
- loss of appetite
- heartburn

In more advanced stages of gastric cancer, the following signs and symptoms may occur:

- blood in the stool
- vomiting
- weight loss for no known reason
- stomach pain
- jaundice (yellowing of eyes and skin)
- ascites (build-up of fluid in the abdomen)
- trouble swallowing

Check with your doctor if you have any of these problems.

# Diagnosis Test

The following tests and procedures may be used:

- physical exam and history
- blood chemistry studies
- complete blood count (CBC)
- upper endoscopy
- barium swallow
- CT scan (CAT scan)
- biopsy

## Prognosis And Treatment Options

The prognosis (chance of recovery) and treatment options depend on the following:

- The stage of the cancer (whether it is in the stomach only or has spread to lymph nodes or other places in the body).

- The patient's general health.

When gastric cancer is found very early, there is a better chance of recovery. Gastric cancer is often in an advanced stage when it is diagnosed. At later stages, gastric cancer can be treated but rarely can be cured.

## Treatment Option Overview

- There are different types of treatment for patients with gastric cancer.

- Five types of standard treatment are used:

  - Surgery

  - Chemotherapy

  - Radiation therapy

  - Chemoradiation

  - Targeted therapy

- New types of treatment are being tested in clinical trials.

- Patients may want to think about taking part in a clinical trial.

- Patients can enter clinical trials before, during, or after starting their cancer treatment.

- Follow-up tests may be needed.

# Part Four
## Other Health Concerns Related To Tobacco Use

# Chapter 35

# Health Effects Of Smoking

## Health Effects Associated With Smoking

Smoking causes harmful effects in various parts of the human body such as organs, blood, muscles, bones, DNA, and the immune system. The changes observed in the human body due to smoking and the reversal effects after quitting are discussed below.

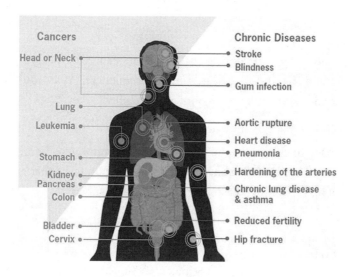

***Figure 35.1.*** Health Effects Of Smoking

About This Chapter: This chapter includes text excerpted from "Health Effects," Smokefree.gov, U.S. Department of Health and Human Services (HHS), June 20, 2012. Reviewed December 2016.

## Brain

### Now

#### Addiction wired

In adolescence, your brain is still "under construction"—as a result, it responds differently to the effects of nicotine than the adult brain. Nicotine is the drug in cigarettes (and other forms of tobacco) that produces addiction. Like heroin and cocaine, nicotine acts on the brain's "reward pathways" to create feelings of satisfaction and pleasure. The developing brain is highly sensitive to the addictive properties of nicotine. Many teens show signs of addiction even at low levels of tobacco use. Exposure to nicotine during adolescence may alter brain development, rewiring the brain for addiction.

#### Brain damage

Smoking can damage your developing brain by stunting the growth of the prefrontal cortex, the part of the brain responsible for "executive" functions (like impulse control and weighing the consequences of your actions). This can alter your ability to make rational decisions about your health, like the decision to quit smoking.

### Later

#### Become addicted

Exposing the brain to nicotine during the teen years can cause permanent changes in the way the brain works and responds to rewards and consequences. As an adult, you may be more susceptible to other addictions (like to alcohol and drugs).

#### Memory problems

Adults with damage to the prefrontal cortex caused by smoking often have problems with attention and memory. They may also have trouble with certain tasks that are necessary to succeed at their job, such as planning, reasoning, and problem-solving.

### Quit

#### Broken addiction cycle

Quitting smoking can re-wire your brain and help break the cycle of addiction. The large number of nicotine receptors in your brain will return to normal levels after about a month of being quit.

#### Fully developed brain

During the teenage years your brain is in a critical development period. Brain development isn't complete until around the age 25. Quitting smoking now will allow your prefrontal cortex to develop normally, and set you up for success as an adult.

## Head And Face

*Now*

### Nerve damage

The hearing nerve pathways aren't fully developed in teens. Exposure to the toxic chemicals in smoke may cause permanent damage to these nerve pathways and set you up for hearing loss later in life. Nicotine restricts the production of rhodopsin, a chemical pigment necessary for night vision. This can make driving at night dangerous.

### Dirty mouth

Smoking dulls the taste buds on your tongue. You may have to put extra salt or hot sauce on your food to make it taste good. Smoking also irritates the lining of the mouth, which can lead to mouth sores and ulcers. Smoking stains your teeth yellow, and gives you nasty bad breath that can't be covered up with gum.

> Short-term use of spit tobacco can cause cracked lips, white spots, sores, and bleeding in the mouth.
>
> *(Source: "Smoking And Tobacco Use," Centers for Disease Control and Prevention (CDC), February 2, 2016.)*

### Zits

The combination of stress and smoking can cause you to breakout and have more zits that last longer.

*Later*

### Hearing loss

Smoking also reduces the oxygen supply to the cochlea, a snail-shaped organ in the inner ear. This results in permanent damage to the cochlea and mild to moderate hearing loss.

### Blindness

Over time, smoking causes physical changes in the eyes that can threaten your eyesight. Smoking increases your risk of developing cataracts and macular degeneration (both can lead to blindness).

### Cavities

Smoking takes a toll on your mouth. Smokers have more oral health problems than non-smokers. You are more likely to have cavities and lose your teeth at a younger age. You are also more likely to get cancers of the mouth and throat.

**Smoker's face**

Over time, smoking can cause your skin to be dry and lose elasticity, leading to wrinkles and stretch marks. Your skin tone may become dull and grayish. By your early 30's, wrinkles will probably begin to appear around your mouth and eyes, adding years to your face.

> Surgery to remove oral cancers caused by tobacco use can lead to serious changes in the face.
>
> *(Source: "Smoking And Tobacco Use," Centers for Disease Control and Prevention (CDC), February 2, 2016.)*

## Quit

**Sharp hearing**

Quitting smoking will keep your hearing sharp. Remember, even mild hearing loss can cause problems (like not clearly hearing homework instructions and doing them wrong).

**Better vision**

Quitting smoking will improve your night vision and help preserve your overall vision by stopping the damage that smoking does to your eyes.

**Clean mouth**

Nobody likes a dirty mouth After a few days without cigarettes, your smile will be brighter and your tastebuds will kick back in. Quitting smoking now will keep your mouth healthy and kissable for years to come.

**Clear skin**

Quitting smoking is better than any zit cream or anti-aging lotion! It can help clear up your skin, and protect it from premature aging and wrinkling.

## Heart

### Now

**Stressed heart**

Smoking raises your blood pressure and puts stress on your heart. Teens who smoke show signs of heart stress, including physical changes to the heart muscle itself, and a higher resting heart rate. These are warning signs that the heart is working too hard.

**Sticky blood**

Smoking makes your blood thick and sticky. The stickier your blood, the harder your heart must work to move it around your body. This puts stress on your heart. Sticky blood is also more likely to form deadly blood clots that block blood flow to your heart, brain, and legs. If you are on the birth control pill, or other hormonal methods of birth control (like the pill, patch, or vaginal ring), your risk for blood clots is even higher.

**Fatty deposits**

Smoking increases the amount of cholesterol and unhealthy fats circulating in the blood. This can lead to fatty deposits on the walls of the arteries, the vessels that carry blood from the heart to the rest of the body. Fatty streaks can often be seen on the artery walls of teens who smoke. This is an early sign of heart disease.

## Later

**Weak heart**

Over time, stress on the heart can weaken it, making it less able to pump oxygenated blood to other parts of your body. Carbon monoxide from the inhaled cigarette smoke also contributes to a lack of oxygen, making the heart work even harder. This increases the risk of heart disease, including heart attacks.

> Nicotine narrows your blood vessels and puts added strain on your heart.
>
> *(Source: "Smoking And Tobacco Use," Centers for Disease Control and Prevention (CDC), February 2, 2016.)*

**Heart attack/stroke**

Over time, thick, sticky blood damages the delicate lining of your blood vessels. This damage can increase your risk for a heart attack or stroke.

**Foot amputation**

Over time, cholesterol, fats and other debris build up on the walls of your arteries. This build-up narrows the arteries and blocks normal blood flow to the heart, brain, and legs. Blocked blood flow to the heart or brain can cause a heart attack or stroke. Blockage in the blood vessels of your legs could result in the amputation of your toes or feet.

## Quit

### Decreased heart risks

Smoking is the leading cause of heart attacks and heart disease. But many of these heart risks can be reversed simply by quitting smoking. Quitting can lower your blood pressure and heart rate almost immediately. Your risk of a heart attack declines within 24 hours.

### Thin blood

When you quit smoking, your blood will become thinner and less likely to form dangerous blood clots. Your heart will also have less work to do, since it will be able to move the blood around your body more easily.

### Lower cholesterol

Quitting smoking will not get rid of the fatty deposits that are already there. But it will lower the levels of cholesterol and fats circulating in your blood, which will help to slow the build up of new fatty deposits in your arteries.

## Lungs

### Now

### Short of breath

Smoking causes inflammation in the small airways and tissues of your lungs. Inflammation can make your chest feel tight, cause you to wheeze, or feel short of breath.

> Smokers suffer shortness of breath (gasp!) almost 3 times more often than nonsmokers.
>
> *(Source: "Smoking And Tobacco Use," Centers for Disease Control and Prevention (CDC), February 2, 2016.)*

### Dead alveoli

Smoking destroys the tiny air sacs, or alveoli, in the lungs that allow oxygen exchange. When you smoke, you are damaging some of those air sacs. Alveoli don't grow back, so when you destroy them you have permanently destroyed part of your lungs.

### Smaller lungs

Teen lungs are still growing; smoking when you're a teen can stunt the growth of your lungs. Teens who smoke have smaller, weaker lungs than teens that don't smoke.

### Dead cilia

Your airways are lined with tiny brush like hairs, called cilia. As air is inhaled, the cilia move back and forth, sweeping out mucus and dirt so your lungs stay clear. Smoking temporarily paralyzes and even kills cilia.

## Later

### Scarred lung

Continued inflammation builds up scar tissue, which leads to permanent scarring of your lung tissue and airways. The scar tissue causes physical changes to your lungs and airways that can make breathing hard. Years of lung irritation can give you a chronic cough with mucus.

### Emphysema

When enough alveoli are destroyed, the disease emphysema develops. Emphysema causes severe shortness of breath, because lungs can no longer exchange oxygen. Emphysema gets worse over time if you continue to smoke. You could end up on oxygen or die due to the development of chronic obstructive pulmonary disease (COPD).

### Stunted lungs

If you smoke as a teen, your lungs may never be able to grow to their full capacity. Smaller lung capacity makes it harder to exercise. You will get tired more easily. And as an adult, you may experience earlier aging of your lungs.

### Respiratory infections

When you smoke your body makes more mucus and the cilia can no longer clear your lungs. This makes you more at risk for infection. Smokers get more colds and respiratory infections than non-smokers.

## Quit

### Stop lung damage

Scarring of the lungs is not reversible. That is why it is important to quit when you are young, before you do permanent damage to your lungs.

### Prevent emphysema

There is no cure for emphysema. But quitting when you are young, before you have done years of damage to the delicate air sacs in your lungs, will help protect you from developing emphysema later.

**Fully developed lungs**

Quitting smoking at any age is beneficial, but quitting now will allow your growing lungs to reach their full capacity. This will help you be a healthier and more physically fit adult.

**Return of cilia**

Cilia start to re-grow and regain normal function very quickly after you quit smoking. They are one of the first things in your body to heal. People sometimes notice that they cough more than usual when they first quitting smoking. This is a sign that the cilia are coming back to life.

## Deoxyribonucleic Acid (DNA)

Now

**Damaged DNA**

Your body is made up of cells, containing genetic material, or DNA, that act as an "instruction manual" for cell growth and function. Every single puff of a cigarette causes damage to DNA. When DNA is damaged, the "instruction manual" gets messed up and the cell can begin growing out of control and create a cancer tumor.

Later

**Cancer**

The damage smoking does to your DNA adds up. Your body tries to repair the damage that smoking does to your DNA, but over time smoking can wear down this repair system and lead to cancer (like lung cancer, pancreatic cancer, stomach cancer, and cancers of the mouth, throat, esophagus and sinuses). In fact, one-third of all cancer deaths are caused by tobacco.

Quit

**Lower cancer risk**

Quitting smoking will prevent new DNA damage from happening, and can even help repair the damage that has already been done. Although quitting smoking at any age is beneficial, quitting when you are young is one of the best ways to lower your risk of getting cancer in the future.

## Stomach And Hormones

Now

### More belly fat

Teens who smoke have more belly fat than non-smokers. Belly fat increases your chances of getting Type 2 Diabetes. It also makes it harder to control diabetes if you already have it.

### Lower estrogen levels

Smoking lowers a female's level of estrogen. Low estrogen levels can cause dry skin, thinning hair, and memory problems.

Later

### Bigger belly

Adults who smoke have bigger bellies and less muscle than non-smokers. And they're more likely to develop Type 2 Diabetes, even if they don't smoke every day. Diabetes is a serious disease that can lead to blindness, heart disease, kidney failure, nerve damage, and amputations.

### Harder to get pregnant

Adult women who smoke have a harder time getting pregnant and having a healthy baby. Smoking can also lead to early menopause, which increases your risk of developing certain diseases (like heart disease, ovarian cancer and osteoporosis).

Quit

### Smaller belly

Quitting smoking will reduce your belly fat and lower your risk of diabetes. If you already have diabetes, quitting can help you keep your blood sugar levels in check.

### Normal estrogen levels

Quitting smoking will help you be a healthy woman now and later. Your estrogen levels will gradually return to normal after you quit smoking. And if you hope to have children someday, quitting smoking right now will increase your chances of a healthy pregnancy in the future.

## Erectile Dysfunction

### Now

**Failure to launch**

Smoking increases the risk of erectile dysfunction or impotence—the inability to achieve or maintain an erection. Tar and chemicals in cigarette smoke cause damage to the blood vessels and arteries that deliver blood to the penis. Without adequate blood flow, the penis can't get or stay hard. Smoking also raises your blood pressure, which can restrict blood flow to the penis.

### Later

**Difficulty having kids**

Toxins from cigarette smoke can damage the genetic material in sperm. Males who smoke have more damaged sperm than males who don't. Damaged sperm can cause infertility or genetic defects problems in their children. Smoking is also associated with having a low sperm count and having sperm that are "poor swimmers" which can further reduce the odds of having a child.

### Quit

**Sexual healing**

If you quit smoking now, you can lower your chances of erectile dysfunction and improve your chances of having a healthy sexual life as an adult.

## Blood And The Immune System

### Now

**High white blood cell count**

When you smoke, the number of white blood cells (a.k.a. the cells that defend your body against infectious disease and foreign materials) stays high. This is a sign that your body is under stress—constantly fighting against the inflammation and damage caused by tobacco. A high white blood cell count is like an SOS from your body, letting you know that you have been injured.

**Longer to heal**

Nutrients, minerals, and oxygen are all supplied to the tissue via the bloodstream. Nicotine causes blood vessels to constrict, which decreases the levels of nutrients supplied to wounds. As a result, wounds take longer to heal.

**Weaker immune system**

Cigarette smoke contains high levels of tar and other chemicals, which can make your immune system less effective at fighting off infections. This means you are more likely to get sick and miss out on things that you want to do.

## Later

**Damage to heart/lungs**

If you continue to smoke as an adult, your white blood cell count will stay abnormally high from the repeated smoking "injuries" to your heart, blood vessels, lungs, and other important organs. White blood cells counts that stay elevated for a long time are linked with an increased risk of heart attacks, strokes, and cancer.

**Painful skin ulcers**

Slow wound healing increases the risk of infection, after an injury or surgery. Painful skin ulcers can develop if adequate blood flow fails to reach skin tissues, causing the tissue to slowly die.

**Arthritis**

Continued weakening of the immune system can make you more vulnerable to auto-immune diseases like rheumatoid arthritis. You may experience serious complications from viruses like the flu. It also decreases your body's ability to fight off cancer!

## Quit

**Normal white blood cell count**

When you quit smoking, your body will begin to heal from the injuries that smoking caused. Eventually, your white blood cell counts will return to normal and will no longer be on the defensive.

**Proper healing**

Quitting smoking will improve blood flow to wounds, allowing important nutrients, minerals, and oxygen to reach the wound and help it heal properly.

**Stronger immune system**

When you quit smoking, your immune system is no longer exposed to tar and other chemicals. It will become stronger, and you will be less likely to get sick.

## Muscles And Bones

### Now

**Tired muscles**

When you smoke, less blood and oxygen flow to your muscles. This makes it harder to build muscle. The lack of oxygen also makes muscles tire more easily.

**Disrupted bone growth**

Your skeleton grows rapidly during your teen years. Bones must constantly form new bone tissue to stay strong and healthy. Ingredients in cigarette smoke disrupt the natural cycle of bone health. Your body is less able to form healthy new bone tissue, and existing bone tissue breaks down more rapidly.

### Later

**Muscle deterioration**

Smokers have more muscle aches and pains than non-smokers. Also, smoking accelerates the breakdown of muscle tissue. Over time, muscle deterioration can lead to weakness and loss of muscle function.

**More broken bones**

Over time, smoking leads to a thinning of bone tissue and loss of bone density. This causes bones to become weak and brittle. Compared to non-smokers, smokers have a higher risk of bone fractures, and their broken bones take longer to heal.

### Quit

**Strong muscles**

Quitting smoking will help increase the availability of oxygen in your blood, and your muscles will become stronger and healthier.

**Stronger bones**

Taking care of your bones during your teen years builds the foundation for healthy bones for the rest of your life. Quitting smoking can reduce your risk of fractures, both now and later in life. Keep your bones strong and healthy by quitting now.

# Chapter 36

# Aneurysms

## What Is An Aneurysm?

An aneurysm is a balloon-like bulge in an artery. Arteries are blood vessels that carry oxygen-rich blood to your body.

Arteries have thick walls to withstand normal blood pressure. However, certain medical problems, genetic conditions, and trauma can damage or injure artery walls. The force of blood pushing against the weakened or injured walls can cause an aneurysm.

An aneurysm can grow large and rupture (burst) or dissect. A rupture causes dangerous bleeding inside the body. A dissection is a split in one or more layers of the artery wall. The split causes bleeding into and along the layers of the artery wall.

Both rupture and dissection often are fatal.

## Types Of Aneurysms

### Aortic Aneurysms

The two types of aortic aneurysm are abdominal aortic aneurysm and thoracic aortic aneurysm. Some people have both types.

### Abdominal Aortic Aneurysms

An aneurysm that occurs in the abdominal portion of the aorta is called an abdominal aortic aneurysm (AAA). Most aortic aneurysms are AAAs.

About This Chapter: This chapter includes text excerpted from "Aneurysm," National Heart, Lung, and Blood Institute (NHLBI), April 1, 2011. Reviewed December 2016.

These aneurysms are found more often now than in the past because of computed tomography scans, or CT scans, done for other medical problems.

Small AAAs rarely rupture. However, AAAs can grow very large without causing symptoms. Routine checkups and treatment for an AAA can help prevent growth and rupture.

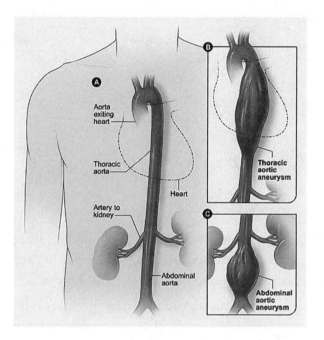

**Figure 36.1.** Aortic Aneurysms

*Figure A shows a normal aorta. Figure B shows a thoracic aortic aneurysm, which is located behind the heart. Figure C shows an abdominal aortic aneurysm, which is located below the arteries that supply blood to the kidneys.*

## Thoracic Aortic Aneurysms

An aneurysm that occurs in the chest portion of the aorta (above the diaphragm, a muscle that helps you breathe) is called a thoracic aortic aneurysm (TAA).

TAAs don't always cause symptoms, even when they're large. Only half of all people who have TAAs notice any symptoms. TAAs are found more often now than in the past because of chest CT scans done for other medical problems.

With a common type of TAA, the walls of the aorta weaken and a section close to the heart enlarges. As a result, the valve between the heart and the aorta can't close properly. This allows blood to leak back into the heart.

A less common type of TAA can develop in the upper back, away from the heart. A TAA in this location may result from an injury to the chest, such as from a car crash.

## Other Types Of Aneurysms

### Brain Aneurysms

Aneurysms in the arteries of the brain are called cerebral aneurysms or brain aneurysms. Brain aneurysms also are called berry aneurysms because they're often the size of a small berry.

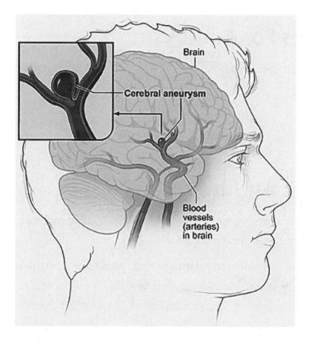

***Figure 36.2.*** Brain Aneurysms

*The illustration shows a typical location of a brain aneurysm in the arteries that supply blood to the brain. The inset image shows a closeup view of the sac-like aneurysm.*

Most brain aneurysms cause no symptoms until they become large, begin to leak blood, or rupture (burst). A ruptured brain aneurysm can cause a stroke.

### Peripheral Aneurysms

Aneurysms that occur in arteries other than the aorta and the brain arteries are called peripheral aneurysms. Common locations for peripheral aneurysms include the popliteal, femoral, and carotid arteries.

The popliteal arteries run down the back of the thighs, behind the knees. The femoral arteries are the main arteries in the groin. The carotid arteries are the two main arteries on each side of your neck.

Peripheral aneurysms aren't as likely to rupture or dissect as aortic aneurysms. However, blood clots can form in peripheral aneurysms. If a blood clot breaks away from the aneurysm, it can block blood flow through the artery.

If a peripheral aneurysm is large, it can press on a nearby nerve or vein and cause pain, numbness, or swelling.

## Other Names For Aneurysm

- Abdominal aortic aneurysm
- Aortic aneurysm
- Berry aneurysm
- Brain aneurysm
- Cerebral aneurysm
- Peripheral aneurysm
- Thoracic aortic aneurysm

## What Causes An Aneurysm?

The force of blood pushing against the walls of an artery combined with damage or injury to the artery's walls can cause an aneurysm.

Many conditions and factors can damage and weaken the walls of the aorta and cause aortic aneurysms. Examples include aging, smoking, high blood pressure, and atherosclerosis. Atherosclerosis is the hardening and narrowing of the arteries due to the buildup of a waxy substance called plaque.

Rarely, infections—such as untreated syphilis (a sexually transmitted infection)—can cause aortic aneurysms. Aortic aneurysms also can occur as a result of diseases that inflame the blood vessels, such as vasculitis.

A family history of aneurysms also may play a role in causing aortic aneurysms.

In addition to the factors above, certain genetic conditions may cause thoracic aortic aneurysms (TAAs). Examples of these conditions include Marfan syndrome, Loeys-Dietz syndrome, Ehlers-Danlos syndrome (the vascular type), and Turner syndrome.

These genetic conditions can weaken the body's connective tissues and damage the aorta. People who have these conditions tend to develop aneurysms at a younger age than other people. They're also at higher risk for rupture and dissection.

Trauma, such as a car accident, also can damage the walls of the aorta and lead to TAAs.

Researchers continue to look for other causes of aortic aneurysms. For example, they're looking for genetic mutations (changes in the genes) that may contribute to or cause aneurysms.

## Who Is At Risk For An Aneurysm?

Certain factors put you at higher risk for an aortic aneurysm. These factors include:

- Male gender. Men are more likely than women to have aortic aneurysms.

- Age. The risk for abdominal aortic aneurysms increases as you get older. These aneurysms are more likely to occur in people who are aged 65 or older.

- Smoking. Smoking can damage and weaken the walls of the aorta.

- A family history of aortic aneurysms. People who have family histories of aortic aneurysms are at higher risk for the condition, and they may have aneurysms before the age of 65.

- A history of aneurysms in the arteries of the legs.

- Certain diseases and conditions that weaken the walls of the aorta. Examples include high blood pressure and atherosclerosis.

Having a bicuspid aortic valve can raise the risk of having a thoracic aortic aneurysm. A bicuspid aortic valve has two leaflets instead of the typical three.

Car accidents or trauma also can injure the arteries and increase the risk for aneurysms.

If you have any of these risk factors, talk with your doctor about whether you need screening for aneurysms.

## What Are The Signs And Symptoms Of An Aneurysm?

The signs and symptoms of an aortic aneurysm depend on the type and location of the aneurysm. Signs and symptoms also depend on whether the aneurysm has ruptured (burst) or is affecting other parts of the body.

Aneurysms can develop and grow for years without causing any signs or symptoms. They often don't cause signs or symptoms until they rupture, grow large enough to press on nearby body parts, or block blood flow.

# How Is An Aneurysm Diagnosed?

If you have an aortic aneurysm but no symptoms, your doctor may find it by chance during a routine physical exam. More often, doctors find aneurysms during tests done for other reasons, such as chest or abdominal pain.

If you have an abdominal aortic aneurysm (AAA), your doctor may feel a throbbing mass in your abdomen. A rapidly growing aneurysm about to rupture (burst) can be tender and very painful when pressed. If you're overweight or obese, it may be hard for your doctor to feel even a large AAA.

If you have an AAA, your doctor may hear rushing blood flow instead of the normal whooshing sound when listening to your abdomen with a stethoscope.

## Specialists Involved

Your primary care doctor may refer you to a cardiothoracic or vascular surgeon for diagnosis and treatment of an aortic aneurysm.

A cardiothoracic surgeon does surgery on the heart, lungs, and other organs and structures in the chest, including the aorta. A vascular surgeon does surgery on the aorta and other blood vessels, except those of the heart and brain.

## Diagnostic Tests And Procedures

To diagnose and study an aneurysm, your doctor may recommend one or more of the following tests.

### Ultrasound And Echocardiography

Ultrasound and echocardiography (echo) are simple, painless tests that use sound waves to create pictures of the structures inside your body. These tests can show the size of an aortic aneurysm, if one is found.

### Computed Tomography Scan

A computed tomography scan, or CT scan, is a painless test that uses X-rays to take clear, detailed pictures of your organs.

During the test, your doctor will inject dye into a vein in your arm. The dye makes your arteries, including your aorta, visible on the CT scan pictures.

Your doctor may recommend this test if he or she thinks you have an AAA or a thoracic aortic aneurysm (TAA). A CT scan can show the size and shape of an aneurysm. This test provides more detailed pictures than an ultrasound or echo.

## Magnetic Resonance Imaging

Magnetic resonance imaging (MRI) uses magnets and radio waves to create pictures of the organs and structures in your body. This test works well for detecting aneurysms and pinpointing their size and exact location.

## Angiography

Angiography is a test that uses dye and special X-rays to show the insides of your arteries. This test shows the amount of damage and blockage in blood vessels.

Aortic angiography shows the inside of your aorta. The test may show the location and size of an aortic aneurysm.

# How Is An Aneurysm Treated?

Aortic aneurysms are treated with medicines and surgery. Small aneurysms that are found early and aren't causing symptoms may not need treatment. Other aneurysms need to be treated.

The goals of treatment may include:

- Preventing the aneurysm from growing

- Preventing or reversing damage to other body structures

- Preventing or treating a rupture or dissection

- Allowing you to continue doing your normal daily activities

Treatment for an aortic aneurysm is based on its size. Your doctor may recommend routine testing to make sure an aneurysm isn't getting bigger. This method usually is used for aneurysms that are smaller than 5 centimeters (about 2 inches) across.

How often you need testing (for example, every few months or every year) is based on the size of the aneurysm and how fast it's growing. The larger it is and the faster it's growing, the more often you may need to be checked.

## Medicines

If you have an aortic aneurysm, your doctor may prescribe medicines before surgery or instead of surgery. Medicines are used to lower blood pressure, relax blood vessels, and lower the risk that the aneurysm will rupture (burst). Beta blockers and calcium channel blockers are the medicines most commonly used.

## Surgery

Your doctor may recommend surgery if your aneurysm is growing quickly or is at risk of rupture or dissection.

The two main types of surgery to repair aortic aneurysms are open abdominal or open chest repair and endovascular repair.

1. Open abdominal or open chest repair

2. Endovascular repair

# How Can An Aneurysm Be Prevented?

The best way to prevent an aortic aneurysm is to avoid the factors that put you at higher risk for one. You can't control all aortic aneurysm risk factors, but lifestyle changes can help you lower some risks.

For example, if you smoke, try to quit. Talk with your doctor about programs and products that can help you quit smoking. Also, try to avoid secondhand smoke.

Another important lifestyle change is following a healthy diet. A healthy diet includes a variety of fruits, vegetables, and whole grains. It also includes lean meats, poultry, fish, beans, and fat-free or low-fat milk or milk products. A healthy diet is low in saturated fat, trans fat, cholesterol, sodium (salt), and added sugar.

Be as physically active as you can. Talk with your doctor about the amounts and types of physical activity that are safe for you.

Work with your doctor to control medical conditions such as high blood pressure and high blood cholesterol. Follow your treatment plans and take all of your medicines as your doctor prescribes.

# Chapter 37
# Asthma

Nearly all tobacco use begins during youth and progresses during young adulthood. More than 3,200 children age 18 or younger smoke their first cigarette every day. Nearly 9 out of 10 smokers start before the age of 18 and almost all start smoking by age 26. Every adult who dies early because of smoking is replaced by two new young smokers. If smoking continues at current rates, 5.6 million—or 1 out of every 13—of today's children will ultimately die prematurely from a smoking-related illness.

Smoking by youth and young adults can cause serious and potentially deadly health issues immediately and into adulthood. Cigarette smoking also causes children and teens to be short of breath and to have less stamina, both of which can affect athletic performance and other physically active pursuits.

## What Is Asthma?

Asthma is a chronic disease that affects the airways of the lungs. During an asthma attack, airways (tubes that carry air to your lungs) become swollen, making it hard to breathe. As the walls of the airways swell, they narrow, and less air gets in and out of the lungs. Cells in the airways can make more mucus (a sticky, thick liquid) than usual, which can make breathing even harder.

About This Chapter: Text in this chapter begins with excerpts from "Smoking And Youth," Centers for Disease Control and Prevention (CDC), October 15, 2014; Text beginning with the heading "What Is Asthma?" is excerpted from "Asthma And Secondhand Smoke," Centers for Disease Control and Prevention (CDC), September 1, 2015; Text under the heading "Asthma Statistics" is excerpted from "Asthma," Centers for Disease Control and Prevention (CDC), October 5, 2015; Text under the heading "Asthma And Absenteeism" is excerpted from "Managing Asthma In The School Environment," U.S. Environmental Protection Agency (EPA), September 8, 2016.

Symptoms of an asthma attack include:

- coughing

- shortness of breath or trouble breathing

- wheezing

- tightness or pain in the chest

Asthma attacks can be mild, moderate, or serious—and even life threatening.

# How Is Smoking Related To Asthma?

If you have asthma, an asthma attack can occur when something irritates your airways and "triggers" an attack. Your triggers might be different from other people's triggers.

Tobacco smoke is one of the most common asthma triggers. Tobacco smoke—including secondhand smoke—is unhealthy for everyone, especially people with asthma. Secondhand smoke is a mixture of gases and fine particles that includes:

- Smoke from a burning cigarette, cigar, or pipe tip

- Smoke that has been exhaled (breathed out) by someone who smokes

Secondhand smoke contains more than 7,000 chemicals, including hundreds that are toxic and about 70 that can cause cancer.

If you have asthma, it's important that you avoid exposure to secondhand smoke.

If you are among the 21 percent of U.S. adults who have asthma and smoke, quit smoking.

# How Is Asthma Treated?

There is no cure for asthma. However, to help control your asthma and avoid attacks:

- Take your medicine exactly as your doctor tells you.

- Stay away from things that can trigger an attack.

Everyone with asthma does not take the same medicine. Some medicines can be breathed in, and some can be taken as a pill. There are two kinds of asthma medicines:

- Quick-relief (can help control symptoms of an asthma attack)

- Long-term control (can help you have fewer and milder attacks, but they don't help you while you are having an asthma attack)

# How Can Asthma Attacks Be Prevented?

If you or a family member has asthma, you can manage it with the help of your health-care provider (for example, by taking your medicines exactly as your doctor tells you) and by avoiding triggers. Staying far away from tobacco smoke is one important way to avoid asthma attacks. Some other helpful tips are:

- Do not smoke or allow others to smoke in your home or car. Opening a window does not protect you from smoke.

- If your state still allows smoking in public areas, look for restaurants and other places that do not allow smoking. "No-smoking sections" in the same restaurant with "smoking sections" do not protect adequately from secondhand smoke—even if there is a filter or ventilation system.

- Make sure your schools are tobacco-free. For schools, a tobacco-free campus policy means no tobacco use or advertising on school property is allowed by anyone at any time. This includes off-campus school events.

# Asthma Statistics

## Number Of Visits To A Healthcare Providers Among Children

**Age:** The percentage of children either with or without asthma who visited a healthcare provider three or more times decreased with age. Among children aged 12 through 17, more children with asthma had three or more visits to a healthcare provider(s), whereas more children without asthma had zero to two visits.

**Table 37.1.** Number Of Visits To A Healthcare Providers Among Children

|  | Children with Asthma | | | Children without Asthma | | |
|---|---|---|---|---|---|---|
|  | **No visits** | **1–2 visits** | **3+ visits** | **No visits** | **1–2 visits** | **3+ visits** |
|  | % | % | % | % | % | % |
| 12–17 | 11.1 | 61.8 | 27.1 | 19.2 | 66.5 | 14.3 |

## Healthcare Coverage Among Children

**Age:** Regardless of age, children with asthma (ages 12 through 17 years: 41%) were more likely to have healthcare coverage through Medicaid or CHIP. Children without asthma in the corresponding age groups (64.2%) were more likely to have privately-funded healthcare coverage.

**Table 37.2.** HealthCare Coverage Among Children

| | Children with Asthma | | | Children without Asthma | | |
|---|---|---|---|---|---|---|
| | Medicaid/CHIP | Private/All other healthcare coverage | No healthcare coverage | Medicaid/CHIP | Private/All other healthcare coverage | No healthcare coverage |
| | % | % | % | % | % | % |
| 12–17 | 41 | 54.8 | 4.1 | 29.5 | 64.2 | 6.3 |

## Asthma-Related Missed School Days Among Children Aged 5–17 Years

The percent of children with asthma who reported one or more missed school days in 2013 was significantly lower than in 2003. Poorly controlled asthma may impair a child's ability to attend school, affect his or her academic performance, and cause parents to miss work to care for an ill child.

The number of reported missed school days among children with asthma was 12.4 million in 2003, 10.4 million in 2008, and 13.8 million in 2013.

The percent of children with asthma who reported one or more asthma-related missed school days in 2013 (49%) was significantly lower than the percent in 2003 (61.4%). However, this percentage was similar to the percentage for 2008 (59.6%). The reported missed school days in each year did not differ by age, sex, race or ethnicity, and poverty level.

# Asthma And Absenteeism

Asthma is the leading cause of school absenteeism due to a chronic condition, accounting for nearly 13 million missed school days per year.

Asthma has reached epidemic proportions in the United States, affecting millions of people of all ages and races. An average of one out of every 10 school-age children now has asthma, and the percentage of children with asthma is rising more rapidly in preschool-age children than in any other age group.

Asthma is a leading cause of school absenteeism due to a chronic condition, accounting for nearly 13 million missed school days per year. Asthma also accounts for many nights of interrupted sleep, limits activity and disrupts family and caregiver routines.

Asthma symptoms that are not severe enough to require a visit to an emergency room or to a physician can still be serious enough to prevent a child with asthma from living a fully active life.

Asthma is a long-term, inflammatory disease that causes the airways of the lungs to tighten and constrict, leading to wheezing, breathlessness, chest tightness and coughing. The inflammation also causes the airways of the lungs to become especially sensitive to a variety of asthma triggers. The particular trigger or triggers and the severity of symptoms can differ for each person with asthma.

Because Americans spend up to 90 percent of their time indoors, exposure to indoor allergens and irritants may play a significant role in triggering asthma episodes. Some of the most common asthma triggers found in schools, as well as techniques to mitigate them.

# Chapter 38

# Chronic Obstructive Pulmonary Disease (COPD)

## What Is COPD?

Chronic obstructive pulmonary disease (COPD) refers to a group of diseases that cause airflow blockage and breathing-related problems. COPD includes emphysema; chronic bronchitis; and in some cases, asthma.

With COPD, less air flows through the airways—the tubes that carry air in and out of your lungs—because of one or more of the following:

- The airways and tiny air sacs in the lungs lose their ability to stretch and shrink back.

- The walls between many of the air sacs are destroyed.

- The walls of the airways become thick and inflamed (irritated and swollen).

- The airways make more mucus than usual, which can clog them and block air flow.

In the early stages of COPD, there may be no symptoms, or you may only have mild symptoms, such as:

- A nagging cough (often called "smoker's cough")

- Shortness of breath, especially with physical activity

- Wheezing (a whistling sound when you breathe)

- Tightness in the chest

About This Chapter: This chapter includes text excerpted from "Chronic Obstructive Pulmonary Disease (COPD)," Centers for Disease Control and Prevention (CDC), March 16, 2016.

As the disease gets worse, symptoms may include:

- Having trouble catching your breath or talking

- Blue or gray lips and/or fingernails (a sign of low oxygen levels in your blood)

- Trouble with mental alertness

- A very fast heartbeat

- Swelling in the feet and ankles

- Weight loss

How severe your COPD symptoms are depends on how damaged your lungs are. If you keep smoking, the damage will get worse faster than if you stop smoking. Among 15 million U.S. adults with COPD, 39 percent continue to smoke.

---

Chronic lower respiratory disease, primarily COPD, was the third leading cause of death in the United States in 2014.

In the United States, tobacco smoke is a key factor in the development and progression of COPD,1 although exposure to air pollutants in the home and workplace, genetic factors, and respiratory infections also play a role.

*(Source: "Chronic Obstructive Pulmonary Disease (COPD)," Centers for Disease Control and Prevention (CDC), September 16, 2016.)*

---

# How Is Smoking Related To COPD?

COPD is usually caused by smoking. Smoking accounts for as many as 8 out of 10 COPD-related deaths. However, as many as 1 out of 4 Americans with COPD never smoked cigarettes.

Smoking during childhood and teenage years can slow how lungs grow and develop. This can increase the risk of developing COPD in adulthood.

# How Can COPD Be Prevented?

The best way to prevent COPD is to never start smoking, and if you smoke, quit. Talk with your doctor about programs and products that can help you quit. Also, stay away from second-hand smoke, which is smoke from burning tobacco products, such as cigarettes, cigars, or pipes. Secondhand smoke also is smoke that has been exhaled, or breathed out, by a person smoking.

# How Is COPD Treated?

Treatment of COPD requires a careful and thorough exam by a doctor. Quitting smoking is the most important first step you can take to treat COPD. Avoiding secondhand smoke is also critical. Other lifestyle changes and treatments include one or more of the following:

- For people with COPD who have trouble eating because of shortness of breath or being tired:

  - Following a special meal plan with smaller, more frequent meals

  - Resting before eating

  - Taking vitamins and nutritional supplements

- A broad program that helps improve the well-being of people who have chronic (ongoing) breathing problems and includes the following:

  - Exercise training

  - Nutritional counseling

  - Education on your lung disease or condition and how to manage it

  - Energy-conserving techniques

  - Breathing strategies

  - Psychological counseling and/or group support

- Medicines such as:

  - A bronchodilator to relax the muscles around the airways. This helps open airways and makes breathing easier. Most bronchodilators are taken with a device called an inhaler.

  - A steroid drug you inhale to reduce swelling in the airways.

  - Antibiotics to treat respiratory infections, if appropriate

  - A vaccination during flu season

- Oxygen therapy, which can help people who have severe COPD and low levels of oxygen in their blood to breathe better.

- Surgery for people who have severe symptoms that have not improved with other treatments.

- Lung volume reduction surgery (LVRS): Surgery to remove diseased parts of the lung so healthier lung tissue can work better. LVRS is not a cure for COPD.

- A lung transplant: Surgery in which one or two healthy lungs from a donor are put in the patient's body to replace diseased lungs. A lung transplant is a last resort.

Even though there is no cure for COPD, these lifestyle changes and treatments can help you breathe easier, stay more active, and slow the progress of the disease.

# Chapter 39
# Deep Vein Thrombosis

Deep Vein Thrombosis and Pulmonary Embolism (DVT/PE) are often underdiagnosed and serious, but preventable medical conditions.

Deep vein thrombosis (DVT) is a medical condition that occurs when a blood clot forms in a deep vein. These clots usually develop in the lower leg, thigh, or pelvis, but they can also occur in the arm.

It is important to know about DVT because it can happen to anybody and can cause serious illness, disability, and in some cases, death. The good news is that DVT is preventable and treatable if discovered early.

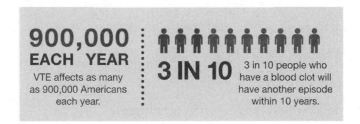

**Figure 39.1.** Blood Clots Affect Many People

## Complications Of DVT

The most serious complication of DVT happens when a part of the clot breaks off and travels through the bloodstream to the lungs, causing a blockage called pulmonary embolism (PE).

About This Chapter: This chapter includes text excerpted from "Venous Thromboembolism (Blood Clots),"
Centers for Disease Control and Prevention (CDC), February 24, 2016.

If the clot is small, and with appropriate treatment, people can recover from PE. However, there could be some damage to the lungs. If the clot is large, it can stop blood from reaching the lungs and is fatal.

In addition, nearly one-third of people who have a DVT will have long-term complications caused by the damage the clot does to the valves in the vein called postthrombotic syndrome (PTS). People with PTS have symptoms such as swelling, pain, discoloration, and in severe cases, scaling or ulcers in the affected part of the body. In some cases, the symptoms can be so severe that a person becomes disabled.

For some people, DVT and PE can become a chronic illness; about 30 percent of people who have had a DVT or PE are at risk for another episode.

# Risk Factors For DVT

Almost anyone can have a DVT. However, certain factors can increase the chance of having this condition. The chance increases even more for someone who has more than one of these factors at the same time.

Following is a list of factors that increase the risk of developing DVT:

- Injury to a vein, often caused by:
  - Fractures,
  - Severe muscle injury, or
  - Major surgery (particularly involving the abdomen, pelvis, hip, or legs)
- Slow blood flow, often caused by:
  - Confinement to bed
  - (e.g., due to a medical condition or after surgery);
  - Limited movement (e.g., a cast on a leg to help heal an injured bone);
  - Sitting for a long time, especially with crossed legs; or
  - Paralysis
- Increased estrogen, often caused by:
  - Birth control pills
  - Hormone replacement therapy, sometimes used after menopause

- Pregnancy, for up to 6 weeks after giving birth
- Certain chronic medical illnesses, such as:
  - Heart disease
  - Lung disease
  - Cancer and its treatment
  - Inflammatory bowel disease (Crohn's disease or ulcerative colitis)
- Other factors that increase the risk of DVT include:
  - Previous DVT or PE
  - Family history of DVT or PE
  - Age (risk increases as age increases)
  - Obesity
  - A catheter located in a central vein
  - Inherited clotting disorders

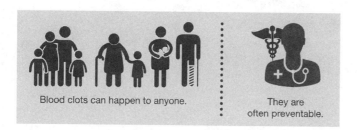

Blood clots can happen to anyone.

They are often preventable.

*Figure 39.2.* Things To Know

# Preventing DVT

The following tips can help prevent DVT:

- Move around as soon as possible after having been confined to bed, such as after surgery, illness, or injury.
- If you're at risk for DVT, talk to your doctor about:
  - Graduated compression stockings (sometimes called "medical compression stockings").
  - Medication (anticoagulants) to prevent DVT.

- When sitting for long periods of time, such as when traveling for more than four hours:

  - Get up and walk around every 2 to 3 hours.

  - Exercise your legs while you're sitting by:

  - Raising and lowering your heels while keeping your toes on the floor

  - Raising and lowering your toes while keeping your heels on the floor

  - Tightening and releasing your leg muscles

  - Wear loose-fitting clothes.

- You can reduce your risk by maintaining a healthy weight, avoiding a sedentary lifestyle, and following your doctor's recommendations based on your individual risk factors.

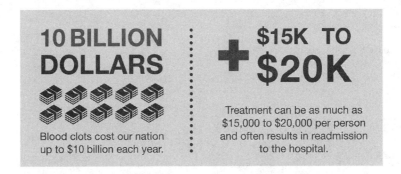

**Figure 39.3.** Blood Clots Are Costly

# Symptoms

## DVT

About half of people with DVT have no symptoms at all. The following are the most common symptoms of DVT that occur in the affected part of the body:

- swelling

- pain

- tenderness

- redness of the skin

If you have any of these symptoms, you should see your doctor as soon as possible.

## Pulmonary Embolism (PE)

You can have a PE without any symptoms of a DVT.

Signs and symptoms of PE can include:

- Difficulty breathing

- Faster than normal or irregular heart beat

- Chest pain or discomfort, which usually worsens with a deep breath or coughing

- Coughing up blood

- Very low blood pressure, lightheadedness, or fainting

If you have any of these symptoms, you should seek medical help immediately.

# Diagnosis Of DVT And PE

The diagnosis of DVT or PE requires special tests that can only be performed by a doctor. That is why it is important for you to seek medical care if you experience any of the symptoms of DVT or PE.

# Treatments For DVT And PE

## DVT

Medication is used to prevent and treat DVT. Compression stockings (also called graduated compression stockings) are sometimes recommended to prevent DVT and relieve pain and swelling. These might need to be worn for 2 years or more after having DVT. In severe cases, the clot might need to be removed surgically.

## PE

Immediate medical attention is necessary to treat PE. In cases of severe, life-threatening PE, there are medicines called thrombolytics that can dissolve the clot. Other medicines, called anticoagulants, may be prescribed to prevent more clots from forming. Some people may need to be on medication long-term to prevent future blood clots.

# Chapter 40
# Digestive Disorders

Smoking affects the entire body, increasing the risk of many life-threatening diseases—including lung cancer, emphysema, and heart disease. Smoking also contributes to many cancers and diseases of the digestive system. Estimates show that about one-fifth of all adults smoke, and each year at least 443,000 Americans die from diseases caused by cigarette smoking.

## What Is The Digestive System?

The digestive system is made up of the gastrointestinal (GI) tract—also called the digestive tract—and the liver, pancreas, and gallbladder. The GI tract is a series of hollow organs joined in a long, twisting tube from the mouth to the anus. The hollow organs that make up the GI tract are the mouth, esophagus, stomach, small intestine, large intestine—which includes the colon and rectum—and anus. Food enters the mouth and passes to the anus through the hollow organs of the GI tract. The liver, pancreas, and gallbladder are the solid organs of the digestive system. The digestive system helps the body digest food, which includes breaking food down into nutrients the body needs. Nutrients are substances the body uses for energy, growth, and cell repair.

About This Chapter: This chapter includes text excerpted from "Smoking And The Digestive System," National Institute of Diabetes and Digestive and Kidney Diseases (NIDDK), September 2013. Reviewed December 2016.

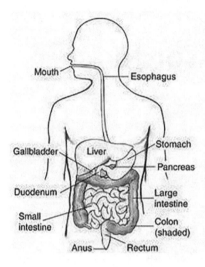

**Figure 40.1.** Digestive System

## Does Smoking Increase The Risk Of Cancers Of The Digestive System?

Smoking has been found to increase the risk of cancers of the

- mouth

- esophagus

- stomach

- pancreas

Research suggests that smoking may also increase the risk of cancers of the

- liver

- colon

- rectum

## What Are The Other Harmful Effects Of Smoking On The Digestive System?

Smoking contributes to many common disorders of the digestive system, such as heartburn and gastroesophageal reflux disease (GERD), peptic ulcers, and some liver diseases. Smoking increases the risk of Crohn's disease, colon polyps, and pancreatitis, and it may increase the risk of gallstones.

## How Does Smoking Affect Heartburn And GERD?

Smoking increases the risk of heartburn and GERD. Heartburn is a painful, burning feeling in the chest caused by reflux, or stomach contents flowing back into the esophagus—the organ that connects the mouth to the stomach. Smoking weakens the lower esophageal sphincter, the muscle between the esophagus and stomach that keeps stomach contents from flowing back into the esophagus. The stomach is naturally protected from the acids it makes to help break down food. However, the esophagus is not protected from the acids. When the lower esophageal sphincter weakens, stomach contents may reflux into the esophagus, causing heartburn and possibly damaging the lining of the esophagus.

GERD is persistent reflux that occurs more than twice a week. Chronic, or long lasting, GERD can lead to serious health problems such as bleeding ulcers in the esophagus, narrowing of the esophagus that causes food to get stuck, and changes in esophageal cells that can lead to cancer.

## How Does Smoking Affect Peptic Ulcers?

Smoking increases the risk of peptic ulcers. Peptic ulcers are sores on the inside lining of the stomach or duodenum, the first part of the small intestine. The two most common causes of peptic ulcers are infection with a bacterium called *Helicobacter pylori (H. pylori)* and long-term use of nonsteroidal anti-inflammatory drugs such as aspirin and ibuprofen.

Researchers are studying how smoking contributes to peptic ulcers. Studies suggest that smoking increases the risk of *H. pylori* infection, slows the healing of peptic ulcers, and increases the likelihood that peptic ulcers will recur. The stomach and duodenum contain acids, enzymes, and other substances that help digest food. However, these substances may also harm the lining of these organs. Smoking has not been shown to increase acid production. However, smoking does increase the production of other substances that may harm the lining, such as pepsin, an enzyme made in the stomach that breaks down proteins. Smoking also decreases factors that protect or heal the lining, including

- blood flow to the lining

- secretion of mucus, a clear liquid that protects the lining from acid

- production of sodium bicarbonate—a salt like substance that neutralizes acid—by the pancreas

The increase in substances that may harm the lining and decrease in factors that protect or heal the lining may lead to peptic ulcers.

## How Does Smoking Affect Liver Disease?

Smoking may worsen some liver diseases, including

- primary biliary cirrhosis, a chronic liver disease that slowly destroys the bile ducts in the liver

- nonalcoholic fatty liver disease (NAFLD), a condition in which fat builds up in the liver

Researchers are still studying how smoking affects primary biliary cirrhosis, NAFLD, and other liver diseases.

Liver diseases may progress to cirrhosis, a condition in which the liver slowly deteriorates and malfunctions due to chronic injury. Scar tissue then replaces healthy liver tissue, partially blocking the flow of blood through the liver and impairing liver functions.

The liver is the largest organ in the digestive system. The liver carries out many functions, such as making important blood proteins and bile, changing food into energy, and filtering alcohol and poisons from the blood. Research has shown that smoking harms the liver's ability to process medications, alcohol, and other toxins and remove them from the body. In some cases, smoking may affect the dose of medication needed to treat an illness.

## How Does Smoking Affect Crohn's Disease?

Current and former smokers have a higher risk of developing Crohn's disease than people who have never smoked.

Crohn's disease is an inflammatory bowel disease that causes irritation in the GI tract. The disease, which typically causes pain and diarrhea, most often affects the lower part of the small intestine; however, it can occur anywhere in the GI tract. The severity of symptoms varies from person to person, and the symptoms come and go. Crohn's disease may lead to complications such as blockages of the intestine and ulcers that tunnel through the affected area into surrounding tissues. Medications may control symptoms. However, many people with Crohn's disease require surgery to remove the affected portion of the intestine.

Among people with Crohn's disease, people who smoke are more likely to

- have more severe symptoms, more frequent symptoms, and more complications

- need more medications to control their symptoms

- require surgery

- have symptoms recur after surgery

The effects of smoking are more pronounced in women with Crohn's disease than in men with the disease.

Researchers are studying why smoking increases the risk of Crohn's disease and makes the disease worse. Some researchers believe smoking might lower the intestines' defenses, decrease blood flow to the intestines, or cause immune system changes that result in inflammation. In people who inherit genes that make them susceptible to developing Crohn's disease, smoking may affect how some of these genes work.

# How Does Smoking Affect Colon Polyps?

People who smoke are more likely to develop colon polyps. Colon polyps are growths on the inside surface of the colon or rectum. Some polyps are benign, or noncancerous, while some are cancerous or may become cancerous.

Among people who develop colon polyps, those who smoke have polyps that are larger, more numerous, and more likely to recur.

# How Does Smoking Affect Pancreatitis?

Smoking increases the risk of developing pancreatitis. Pancreatitis is inflammation of the pancreas, which is located behind the stomach and close to the duodenum. The pancreas secretes digestive enzymes that usually do not become active until they reach the small intestine. When the pancreas is inflamed, the digestive enzymes attack the tissues of the pancreas.

# How Does Smoking Affect Gallstones?

Some studies have shown that smoking may increase the risk of developing gallstones. However, research results are not consistent and more study is needed.

Gallstones are small, hard particles that develop in the gallbladder, the organ that stores bile made by the liver. Gallstones can move into the ducts that carry digestive enzymes from the gallbladder, liver, and pancreas to the duodenum, causing inflammation, infection, and abdominal pain.

## Can The Damage To The Digestive System From Smoking Be Reversed?

Quitting smoking can reverse some of the effects of smoking on the digestive system. For example, the balance between factors that harm and protect the stomach and duodenum lining returns to normal within a few hours of a person quitting smoking. The effects of smoking on how the liver handles medications also disappear when a person stops smoking. However, people who stop smoking continue to have a higher risk of some digestive diseases, such as colon polyps and pancreatitis, than people who have never smoked.

Quitting smoking can improve the symptoms of some digestive diseases or keep them from getting worse. For example, people with Crohn's disease who quit smoking have less severe symptoms than smokers with the disease.

## Eating, Diet, And Nutrition

Eating, diet, and nutrition can play a role in causing, preventing, and treating some of the diseases and disorders of the digestive system that are affected by smoking, including heartburn and GERD, liver diseases, Crohn's disease, colon polyps, pancreatitis, and gallstones.

# Chapter 41

# Eye Disease

## Smoking And Eyesight

Smoking is as bad for your eyes as it is for the rest of your body. If you smoke, you can develop serious eye conditions that can cause vision loss or blindness. Two of the greatest threats to your eyesight are:

- Macular degeneration

- Cataracts

Macular degeneration, also called age-related macular degeneration (AMD), is an eye disease that affects central vision. You need central vision to see objects clearly and for common tasks such as reading, recognizing faces, and driving.

There are two forms of AMD: dry AMD and wet AMD. Macular degeneration always begins in the dry form, and sometimes progresses to the more advanced wet form, where vision loss can be very rapid if untreated.

Cataracts cause blurry vision that worsens over time. Without surgery, cataracts can lead to serious vision loss. The best way to protect your sight from damage linked to smoking is to quit or never start smoking.

## Symptoms Of Eye Diseases Related To Smoking

You may think your eyes are fine, but the only way to know for sure is by getting a full eye exam. AMD often has no early symptoms, so an eye exam is the best way to spot this eye

About This Chapter: This chapter includes text excerpted from "Vision Loss, Blindness, And Smoking," Centers for Disease Control and Prevention (CDC), January 18, 2016.

217

disease early. An eye specialist will place special drops in your eyes to widen your pupils. This offers a better view of the back of your eye, where a thin layer of tissue (the retina) changes light into signals that go to the brain. The macula is a small part of the retina that you need for sharp, central vision.

When symptoms of AMD do occur, they can include:

- Blurred vision or a blurry spot in your central vision

- The need for more light to read or do other tasks

- Straight lines that look wavy

- Trouble recognizing faces

Eye injections are often the preferred treatment for wet AMD. Your doctor can inject a drug to stop the growth of these blood vessels and stop further damage to your eyes. You may need injections on a regular basis to save your vision.

## How Does Smoking Affect Your Eyes?

Smoking causes changes in the eyes that can lead to vision loss. If you smoke:

- You are twice as likely to develop AMD compared with a nonsmoker.

- You are two to three times more likely to develop cataracts compared with a nonsmoker.

## How Can You Prevent Vision Loss Related To Smoking?

If you smoke, stop. Quitting may lower your risk for both AMD and cataracts.

If you already have AMD, quitting smoking may slow the disease. AMD tends to get worse over time. Quitting smoking is something within your control that may help save your sight. Other healthy habits may also help protect your eyes from cataracts and AMD:

- Exercise regularly

- Maintain normal blood pressure and cholesterol levels.

- Eat a healthy diet rich in green, leafy vegetables and fish.

- Wear sunglasses and a hat with a brim to protect your eyes from sunlight.

# How Is A Cataract Treated?

The symptoms of an early cataract may improve with new eyeglasses, brighter lighting, antiglare sunglasses, or magnifying lenses.

When glasses and brighter lighting don't help, you may need surgery. A doctor will remove the cloudy lens and replace it with an artificial lens. This clear, plastic lens becomes a permanent part of your eye.

# Help For Vision Loss

Coping with vision loss can be frightening, but there is help to make the most of the vision you have left and to continue enjoying your friends, family, and special interests. If you've already lost some sight, ask your healthcare professional about low-vision counseling and devices such as high-powered lenses, magnifiers, and talking computers.

# Chapter 42
# Heart Disease And Stroke

## What Is Heart Disease And Stroke?

Heart disease and stroke are cardiovascular (heart and blood vessel) diseases (CVDs).

Heart disease includes several types of heart conditions. The most common type in the United States is coronary heart disease (also known as coronary artery disease), which is narrowing of the blood vessels that carry blood to the heart. This can cause:

- Chest pain

- Heart attack (when blood flow to the heart becomes blocked and a section of the heart muscle is damaged or dies)

- Heart failure (when the heart cannot pump enough blood and oxygen to support other organs)

- Arrhythmia (when the heart beats too fast, too slow, or irregularly)

A stroke occurs when the blood supply to the brain is blocked or when a blood vessel in the brain bursts, causing brain tissue to die. Stroke can cause disability (such as paralysis, muscle weakness, trouble speaking, memory loss) or death.

About This Chapter: This chapter includes text excerpted from "Smoking And Heart Disease And Stroke," Centers for Disease Control and Prevention (CDC), October 13, 2016.

**Smoking And CVD**

Smoking is a major cause of CVD and causes one of every three deaths from CVD. Smoking can:

- Raise triglycerides (a type of fat in your blood)
- Lower "good" cholesterol (HDL)
- Make blood sticky and more likely to clot, which can block blood flow to the heart and brain
- Damage cells that line the blood vessels
- Increase the buildup of plaque (fat, cholesterol, calcium, and other substances) in blood vessels
- Cause thickening and narrowing of blood vessels

# How Is Breathing Secondhand Smoke Related To Heart Disease And Stroke?

Breathing secondhand smoke also harms your health. Secondhand smoke is the smoke from burning tobacco products. Secondhand smoke also is smoke breathed out by a smoker.

Breathing secondhand smoke can cause coronary heart disease, including heart attack and stroke. Know the facts:

- Secondhand smoke causes nearly 34,000 early deaths from coronary heart disease each year in the United States among nonsmokers.

- Nonsmokers who breathe secondhand smoke at home or at work increase their risk of developing heart disease by 25–30 percent. Secondhand smoke increases the risk for stroke by 20–30 percent.

- Each year, secondhand smoke exposure causes more than 8,000 deaths from stroke.

- Breathing secondhand smoke interferes with the normal functioning of the heart, blood, and vascular systems in ways that increase your risk of having a heart attack.

- Even briefly breathing secondhand smoke can damage the lining of blood vessels and cause your blood to become stickier. These changes can cause a deadly heart attack.

# How Can Heart Disease And Stroke Be Prevented?

Heart disease and stroke are major causes of death and disability in the United States. Many people are at high risk for these diseases and don't know it. The good news is that many risk factors for heart disease and stroke can be prevented or controlled.

The federal government's Million Hearts® initiative aims to prevent 1 million heart attacks and strokes by 2017. It's important to know your risk for heart disease and stroke and to take action to reduce that risk. A good place to start is with the ABCS of heart health:

- **A**spirin: Aspirin may help reduce your risk for heart disease and stroke. But do not take aspirin if you think you are having a stroke. It can make some types of stroke worse. Before taking aspirin, talk to your doctor about whether aspirin is right for you.

- **B**lood pressure: Control your blood pressure.

- **C**holesterol: Manage your cholesterol.

- **S**moking: Quit smoking, or don't start.

In addition to your ABCS, several lifestyle choices can help protect your heart and brain health. These include the following:

- Avoid breathing secondhand smoke.

- Eat low-fat, low-salt foods most of the time and fresh fruits and vegetables.

- Maintain a healthy weight.

- Exercise regularly.

- Limit alcohol use.

- Get other health conditions (such as diabetes) under control.

# Chapter 43

# Stress And Depression

## Depression

### What Is Depression?

Depression is more than feeling sad or having a bad day. People with depression usually experience other signs like the following for two weeks or longer:

If these problems are keeping you from participating in your day-to-day activities, you should consider talking to someone you trust about how you're feeling. This person might be a family member, a friend, someone a little older you look up to, or a teacher. They can help you sort through feelings, put things in perspective, or just be there to listen to you vent. They can also help you find ways to get more help like seeing a doctor or therapist. You don't have to tackle this all by yourself.

### Who Gets Depression?

Anyone can get depressed. Depression can happen at any age and to any type of person. But the following types of people seem more likely to get depressed than others:

- Women and girls
- People who smoke
- People with medical problems
- People who are stressed

About This Chapter: This chapter includes text excerpted from "Mood," Smokefree.gov, U.S. Department of Health and Human Services (HHS), December 12, 2011. Reviewed December 2016.

### How Is Depression Different From Withdrawal From Smoking?

Feeling irritable, restless, or down is common after you quit smoking. These are symptoms of withdrawal from nicotine. Changes in mood from quitting smoking usually get better in one or two weeks, and they are not as serious as depression.

If you find that you are feeling down after quitting smoking, then you should talk about this with friends and family and also call your doctor.

### If I Get Depressed After Quitting Smoking, Should I Start Smoking Again?

No. It might be tempting to start again, but you should look for other ways to get help with your depression. Smoking is not a treatment for depression. And remember, smoking is linked to many serious health problems for both the smoker and the people around them. Finding ways to help your depression AND quit smoking is the best way to go.

### Is It Worth Getting Treatment For Depression?

Yes! Treatment almost always helps. Many people think that depression is not real, can't be all that bad, or is a sign that they are simply not tough enough to deal with life. None of these are true. Getting treatment for your depression is definitely worth it.

# Stress

Stress can come from major life events or from daily hassles that add up over time. Dealing with a lot of small stresses can weigh you down and wear you out as much one large event that causes you stress. Some sources of stress for teens include:

- Abuse
- Changes in your body
- Death of a friend or relative
- Family financial problems
- Feeling bad about yourself
- Feeling unsafe
- Illness or family problems
- Moving or changing schools
- Problems with friends or classmates
- Relationship problems

- School demands and frustration
- Separation or divorce of parents
- Taking on too many activities or having too high expectations

## The Stress-Smoking Link

Many teens say that stress is one of the reasons they smoke. Does this sound like you? "Cigarettes help me calm down and relax."

It's important to find ways to handle stress and take care of yourself without smoking. Did you know that most people in the United States are non-smokers? If most other people can cope with stress without cigarettes, you can too.

---

## Remember RAIN

RAIN is a great tool that might help you to better understand and deal with stress in a way that empowers you and is longer lasting that what you get from cigarettes.

- **R**ecognize what is happening: Focus on your thoughts, feelings, and emotions. Notice how your body responds. Is your heart racing? Are you holding your breath? Clenching your teeth?

- **A**llow life to be just as it is: You might want to push away the thoughts and feelings you're having because they're so uncomfortable. Give yourself the OK to feel what you're feeling and think what you're thinking.

- **I**nvestigate inner experience with kindness: Sometimes "Recognize" and "Allow" are enough to relieve some of the stress. Other times you need to dig deeper. Investigating with kindness means exploring more of what you're feeling and sensing—without beating yourself up over it.

- **N**on-identification: Dealing with stress involves a balance between acknowledging what you're experiencing but not connecting that experience with who you are. You are not defined by the things going on around you.

*(Source: "LGBT Smoking," Smokefree.gov, August 11, 2013.)*

---

# Coping

## Ten Ways To Cope And Not Have A Smoke

- Take a time-out.

   A short break from a stressful or upsetting situation can help you think more clearly and make a healthy decision about what to do next.

- Express yourself.

  Text or call a friend to "vent" or talk to an adult who you think will understand how you are feeling.

- Distract yourself.

  Take a walk, play a game, or read a good book.

- Move your body.

  If you are feeling low, take a walk or jog around the block.

- Rehearse and practice dealing with stressful situations.

  If you are nervous about talking to your teacher, practice what you will say in front of a mirror. Got a big performance or game coming up? Picture yourself nailing it!

- Make lists and set short-term goals.

  Break down your large tasks into smaller steps. Then cross off each step as you go to see your progress.

- Don't let negative thoughts take over.

  If you are feeling down about yourself or about life, make a list of things that you are grateful for.

- Give yourself a break.

  Instead of demanding total perfection from yourself, allow yourself to be happy with doing a pretty good job. Just aim to do your best, knowing you don't have to be perfect.

- Exercise, eat regularly, and get plenty of sleep.

  Being physically run down can make it much harder to deal with a bad mood. Take care of yourself.

- When you are feeling extremely upset, use the Stop-Breathe-Think method:

  Take a timeout and stop, think about what's going on, and take a deep breath.

# Chapter 44
# Nicotine Poisoning

Liquid nicotine is manufactured for use in electronic cigarettes (e-cigarettes) and can be highly toxic when exposed in high doses. According to reports, "ingestion or skin exposure to small amounts of such solutions, ranging from one teaspoon to a tablespoon based on body weight and skin morphology, carries with it the potential for serious toxicity or even death."

Liquid nicotine comes in a variety of colors and flavors, like cotton candy, blueberry, and cherry, which can make them attractive to young children. The increased popularity of e-cigarettes in recent years has contributed to a large increase in liquid nicotine exposures. According to the American Association of Poison Control Centers (AAPCC), there were over 3,700 reported exposures to poison centers in 2014. Many types of liquid nicotine containers are currently manufactured without childproof packaging.

Under the Poison Prevention Packaging Act (PPPA), the U.S. Consumer Product Safety Commission (CPSC) has promulgated childproof packaging for numerous consumer products, including over-the-counter medication and household cleaning supplies. The CPSC currently lacks authority under the PPPA to require similar special packaging requirements for liquid nicotine because most liquid nicotine is derived from tobacco and is, consequently, a "tobacco product," which is exclusively regulated by the Food and Drug Administration (FDA).

About This Chapter: Text in this chapter begins with excerpts from "Child Nicotine Poisoning Prevention Act Of 2015," U.S. House of Representatives, January 11, 2016; Text beginning with the heading "Signs And Symptoms" is excerpted from "NICOTINE: Systemic Agent," Centers for Disease Control and Prevention (CDC), May 12, 2011. Reviewed December 2016.

# Signs And Symptoms

- **Time Course:** Nicotine poisoning typically (but not always) produces toxicity in two phases: stimulation/excitation (early) followed quickly by inhibition/depression (late). Some patient/victims may only exhibit late phase effects. Onset of physical effects is dependent on route of exposure. Early phase findings occur within 15 minutes to 1 hour. Vomiting is the most common symptom of nicotine poisoning. Late phase findings occur within 30 minutes to 4 hours. The duration of symptoms is about 1 to 2 hours following mild exposure, and up to 18 to 24 hours following severe exposure. Death may occur within 1 hour after severe exposure.

- **Effects Of Short-Term (LESS Than 8-Hours) Exposure:** At low concentrations, nicotine causes tremor and increases in heart rate, respiratory rate, blood pressure, and level of alertness. More severe exposures cause muscle fasciculations (involuntary twitching), seizures, and abnormal heart rhythms; these effects are followed by multi-system organ depression including slow heart rate (bradycardia), low blood pressure (hypotension), and paralysis of the muscles that control breathing. Vomiting occurs in more then 50 percent of symptomatic patient/victims. Death may occur, and is typically due to paralysis of the muscles that control breathing, a build-up of fluid in the airways (bronchorrhea), and failure of the heart and blood vessels (cardiovascular collapse).

- **Eye Exposure:**

  - Irritation and redness.

  - Pure nicotine in the eye may cause severe pain and inflammation of the conjuctiva.

  - Severe exposure may cause opacification of the cornea.

- **Ingestion Exposure:**

  - Early phase: nausea, vomiting (emesis), abdominal pain, and increased salivation; fluid build-up in the airways (bronchorrhea); rapid, heavy breathing (hyperpnea); high blood pressure (hypertension), rapid heart rate (tachycardia), and generalized narrowing of the blood vessels (vasoconstriction) with pale skin; and headache, dizziness, confusion, agitation, restlessness, loss of balance and difficulty walking, and visual and hearing (auditory) distortions.

  - Late phase: diarrhea (particularly at larger doses); shallow breathing (hypoventilation), no breathing (apnea), low blood pressure (hypotension), slow heart rate (bradycardia), abnormal heart rhythms (dysrhythmias), and shock (critically low blood pressure); and loss of normal reflexes (hyporeflexia), loss of normal muscle tone (hypotonia), lethargy, weakness, paralysis, and coma (long-term loss of consciousness).

- Possible burning sensation in the mouth, throat, and stomach.

- Absorption of nicotine by ingestion is not complete because acid in the stomach prevents nicotine from being very well absorbed.

- **Inhalation Exposure:**

  - See Ingestion Exposure

- **Skin Exposure:**

  - Irritation and redness (erythema)

  - Occupational handling of tobacco leaves may result in green tobacco sickness caused by dermal absorption of nicotine.

  - Absorption through the skin and particularly through the mucous membranes may result in whole-body (systemic) toxicity.

  - Some patient/victims may exhibit an allergic reaction to nicotine.

  - See Ingestion Exposure

# First Aid

- **General Information:** Initial treatment is primarily supportive.

- **Antidote:** Use of atropine is a mainstay of treatment for cholinergic toxicity.

For pediatric patient/victims administer 0.02 mg/kg of atropine intravenously (IV). Repeat as necessary.

For adult patient/victims administer 2 to 3 mg intravenously (IV). Repeat as necessary.

- **Eye:**

  - Immediately remove the patient/victim from the source of exposure.

  - Immediately wash eyes with large amounts of tepid water for at least 15 minutes.

  - Seek medical attention immediately

- **Ingestion:**

  - Immediately remove the patient/victim from the source of exposure.

- Ensure that the patient/victim has an unobstructed airway.

- Do not induce vomiting (emesis).

- Patient/victims often vomit spontaneously.

- Only if airway is secured administer charcoal as a slurry (240 mL water/30 g charcoal). Usual dose: 25 to 100 g in adults/adolescents, 25 to 50 g in children (1 to 12 years), and 1 g/kg in infants less than 1 year old.

- Do not administer antacids; alkaline conditions improve the absorption of nicotine.

- Monitor heart function and evaluate for low blood pressure (hypotension), abnormal heart rhythms (dysrhythmias), and reduced respiratory function (respiratory depression).

- Evaluate for low blood sugar (hypoglycemia), electrolyte disturbances, and low oxygen levels (hypoxia).

- If evidence of shock or low blood pressure (hypotension) is observed, begin intravenous (IV) fluid administration. If fluid administration fails to reverse hypotension, dopamine and norepinephrine may be used.

- If seizures occur, treat them with benzodiazepines.

- Maintain adequate hydration and urine output.

- Seek medical attention immediately

- **Inhalation:**

  - Immediately remove the patient/victim from the source of exposure.

  - Evaluate respiratory function and pulse.

  - Ensure that the patient/victim has an unobstructed airway.

  - Only if the airway is secured, administer charcoal as a slurry (240 mL water/30 g charcoal). Usual dose: 25 to 100 g in adults/adolescents, 25 to 50 g in children (1 to 12 years), and 1 g/kg in infants less than 1 year old.

  - If shortness of breath occurs or breathing is difficult (dyspnea), administer oxygen.

  - Assist ventilation as required. Always use a barrier or bag-valve-mask device.

  - If breathing has ceased (apnea), provide artificial respiration.

- See the Ingestion section for first aid recommendations.

- Seek medical attention immediately

- **Skin:**

  - Immediately remove the patient/victim from the source of exposure.

  - See the Decontamination section for patient/victim decontamination procedures.

  - If signs of systemic exposure develop, see the Ingestion section for first aid recommendations.

  - Seek medical attention immediately

# Who To Contact In An Emergency

In the event of a poison emergency, call the poison center immediately at 1-800-222-1222. If the person who is poisoned cannot wake up, has a hard time breathing, or has convulsions, call 911 emergency services.

# Chapter 45

# Osteoporosis

Many of the health problems caused by tobacco use are well known. Cigarette smoking causes heart disease, lung and esophageal cancer, and chronic lung disease. Additionally, several research studies have identified smoking as a risk factor for osteoporosis and bone fracture. According to the Centers for Disease Control and Prevention (CDC), more than 16 million Americans are living with a disease caused by smoking.

## Facts About Osteoporosis

Osteoporosis is a condition in which bones weaken and are more likely to fracture. Fractures from osteoporosis can result in pain and disability. In the United States, more than 53 million people either already have osteoporosis or are at high risk due to low bone mass.

In addition to smoking, risk factors for developing osteoporosis include:

- thinness or small frame

- family history of the disease

- being postmenopausal and particularly having had early menopause

- abnormal absence of menstrual periods (amenorrhea)

- prolonged use of certain medications, such as those used to treat lupus, asthma, thyroid deficiencies, and seizures

- low calcium intake

About This Chapter: This chapter includes text excerpted from "Smoking And Bone Health," National Institute of Arthritis and Musculoskeletal and Skin Diseases (NIAMS), May 2016.

- lack of physical activity

- excessive alcohol intake

Osteoporosis can often be prevented. It is known as a "silent" disease because, if undetected, bone loss can progress for many years without symptoms until a fracture occurs. It has been called a childhood disease with old age consequences because building healthy bones in youth helps prevent osteoporosis and fractures later in life. However, it is never too late to adopt new habits for healthy bones.

# Smoking And Osteoporosis

Cigarette smoking was first identified as a risk factor for osteoporosis decades ago. Studies have shown a direct relationship between tobacco use and decreased bone density. Analyzing the impact of cigarette smoking on bone health is complicated. It is hard to determine whether a decrease in bone density is due to smoking itself or to other risk factors common among smokers. For example, in many cases smokers are thinner than nonsmokers, tend to drink more alcohol, may be less physically active, and have poor diets. Women who smoke also tend to have an earlier menopause than nonsmokers. These factors place many smokers at an increased risk for osteoporosis apart from their tobacco use.

In addition, studies on the effects of smoking suggest that smoking increases the risk of having a fracture. As well, smoking has been shown to have a negative impact on bone healing after fracture.

# Osteoporosis Management Strategies

**Start by quitting:** The best thing smokers can do to protect their bones is to quit smoking. Smoking cessation, even later in life, may help limit smoking-related bone loss.

**Eat a well-balanced diet rich in calcium and vitamin D:** Good sources of calcium include low-fat dairy products; dark green, leafy vegetables; and calcium-fortified foods and beverages. Supplements can help ensure that you get adequate amounts of calcium each day, especially in people with a proven milk allergy. The Institute of Medicine recommends a daily calcium intake of 1,000 mg (milligrams) for men and women up to age 50. Women over age 50 and men over age 70 should increase their intake to 1,200 mg daily.

Vitamin D plays an important role in calcium absorption and bone health. Food sources of vitamin D include egg yolks, saltwater fish, and liver. Many people, especially those who are older, may need vitamin D supplements to achieve the recommended intake of 600 to 800 IU (International Units) each day.

**Exercise for your bone health:** Like muscle, bone is living tissue that responds to exercise by becoming stronger. Weight-bearing exercise that forces you to work against gravity is the best exercise for bone.

Some examples include walking, climbing stairs, weight training, and dancing. Regular exercise, such as walking, may help prevent bone loss and will provide many other health benefits.

**Avoid excessive use of alcohol:** Chronic alcohol use has been linked to an increase in fractures of the hip, spine, and wrist. Drinking too much alcohol interferes with the balance of calcium in the body. It also affects the production of hormones, which have a protective effect on bone, and of vitamins, which we need to absorb calcium. Excessive alcohol consumption also can lead to more falls and related fractures.

**Talk to your doctor about a bone density test:** A bone mineral density (BMD) test measures bone density at various sites of the body. This safe and painless test can detect osteoporosis before a fracture occurs and can predict one's chances of fracturing in the future. If you are a current or former smoker, you may want to ask your healthcare provider whether you are a candidate for a BMD test, which can help determine whether medication should be considered.

**See if medication is an option for you:** There is no cure for osteoporosis. However, several medications are available to prevent and treat the disease in postmenopausal women and in men. Your doctor can help you decide whether medication might be right for you.

## How Does Smoking Affect My Bones?

Recent studies show a direct relationship between tobacco use and decreased bone density. Smoking is one of many factors—including weight, alcohol consumption, and activity level—that increase your risk for osteoporosis, a condition in which bones weaken and become more likely to fracture.

Significant bone loss has been found in older women and men who smoke. Quitting smoking appears to reduce the risk for low bone mass and fractures. However, it may take several years to lower a former smoker's risk.

In addition, smoking from an early age puts women at even higher risk for osteoporosis. Smoking lowers the level of the hormone estrogen in your body, which can cause you to go through menopause earlier, boosting your risk for osteoporosis.

*(Source: "Effects Of Smoking On Your Health" BeTobaccoFree.gov, November 15, 2012.)*

Chapter 46

# Periodontal Disease

## What Is Periodontal Disease?

Gum (periodontal) disease is an infection of the gums and can affect the bone structure that supports your teeth. In severe cases, it can make your teeth fall out. Smoking is an important cause of severe gum disease in the United States.

Gum disease starts with bacteria (germs) on your teeth that get under your gums. If the germs stay on your teeth for too long, layers of plaque (film) and tartar (hardened plaque) develop. This buildup leads to early gum disease, called gingivitis.

When gum disease gets worse, your gums can pull away from your teeth and form spaces that get infected. This is severe gum disease, also called periodontitis. The bone and tissue that hold your teeth in place can break down, and your teeth may loosen and need to be pulled out.

Need another reason to quit smoking? Smoking is one of the most significant risk factors associated with the development of gum disease. Additionally, smoking can lower the chances for successful treatment.

*(Source: "Periodontal (Gum) Disease: Causes, Symptoms, And Treatments" National Institute of Dental and Craniofacial Research (NIDCR), September 2013.)*

About This Chapter: This chapter includes text excerpted from "Smoking, Gum Disease, And Tooth Loss," Centers for Disease Control and Prevention (CDC), September 1, 2015.

# Warning Signs And Symptoms of Periodontal Disease

- Gums that have pulled away from your teeth
- Loose teeth
- Painful chewing
- Red or swollen gums
- Sensitive teeth
- Tender or bleeding gum

# How Is Smoking Related To Periodontal Disease?

Smoking weakens your body's infection fighters (your immune system). This makes it harder to fight off a gum infection. Once you have gum damage, smoking also makes it harder for your gums to heal.

What does this mean for me if I am a smoker?

- You have twice the risk for gum disease compared with a nonsmoker.
- The more cigarettes you smoke, the greater your risk for gum disease.
- The longer you smoke, the greater your risk for gum disease.
- Treatments for gum disease may not work as well for people who smoke.

Tobacco use in any form—cigarettes, pipes, and smokeless (spit) tobacco—raises your risk for gum disease.

# How Can Periodontal Disease Be Prevented?

You can help avoid gum disease with good dental habits.

- Brush your teeth twice a day.
- Floss often to remove plaque.
- See a dentist regularly for checkups and professional cleanings.
- Don't smoke. If you smoke, quit.

# How Is Periodontal Disease Treated?

Regular cleanings at your dentist's office and daily brushing and flossing can help treat early gum disease (gingivitis).

More severe gum disease may require:

- Deep cleaning below the gum line.

- Prescription mouth rinse or medicine.

- Surgery to remove tartar deep under the gums.

- Surgery to help heal bone or gums lost to periodontitis. Your dentist may use small bits of bone to fill places where bone has been lost. Or your dentist may move tissue from one place in your mouth to cover exposed tooth roots.

If you smoke or use spit tobacco, quitting will help your gums heal after treatment.

# Chapter 47
# Peripheral Arterial Disease

## What Is Peripheral Artery Disease?

Peripheral artery disease (P.A.D.) is a disease in which plaque builds up in the arteries that carry blood to your head, organs, and limbs. Plaque is made up of fat, cholesterol, calcium, fibrous tissue, and other substances in the blood.

When plaque builds up in the body's arteries, the condition is called atherosclerosis. Over time, plaque can harden and narrow the arteries. This limits the flow of oxygen-rich blood to your organs and other parts of your body.

P.A.D. usually affects the arteries in the legs, but it also can affect the arteries that carry blood from your heart to your head, arms, kidneys, and stomach. This chapter focuses on P.A.D. that affects blood flow to the legs.

## Other Names For Peripheral Artery Disease

- Atherosclerotic peripheral arterial disease
- Claudication
- Hardening of the arteries
- Leg cramps from poor circulation
- Peripheral arterial disease
- Peripheral vascular disease

About This Chapter: This chapter includes text excerpted from "Peripheral Artery Disease," National Heart, Lung, and Blood Institute (NHLBI), June 22, 2016.

- Poor circulation

- Vascular disease

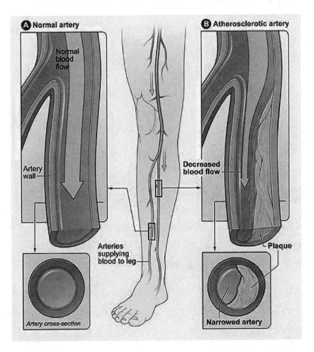

**Figure 47.1.** Normal Artery And Artery With Plaque Buildup

*The illustration shows how P.A.D. can affect arteries in the legs. Figure A shows a normal artery with normal blood flow. The inset image shows a cross-section of the normal artery. Figure B shows an artery with plaque buildup that's partially blocking blood flow. The inset image shows a cross-section of the narrowed artery.*

## What Causes Peripheral Artery Disease?

The most common cause of peripheral artery disease (P.A.D.) is atherosclerosis. Atherosclerosis is a disease in which plaque builds up in your arteries. The exact cause of atherosclerosis isn't known.

The disease may start if certain factors damage the inner layers of the arteries. These factors include:

- Smoking

- High amounts of certain fats and cholesterol in the blood

- High blood pressure

- High amounts of sugar in the blood due to insulin resistance or diabetes

When damage occurs, your body starts a healing process. The healing may cause plaque to build up where the arteries are damaged.

Eventually, a section of plaque can rupture (break open), causing a blood clot to form at the site. The buildup of plaque or blood clots can severely narrow or block the arteries and limit the flow of oxygen-rich blood to your body.

# Who Is At Risk For Peripheral Artery Disease?

Peripheral artery disease (P.A.D.) affects millions of people in the United States. The disease is more common in blacks than any other racial or ethnic group. The major risk factors for P.A.D. are smoking, older age, and having certain diseases or conditions.

## Smoking

Smoking is the main risk factor for P.A.D. and your risk increases if you smoke or have a history of smoking. Quitting smoking slows the progress of P.A.D. People who smoke and people who have diabetes are at highest risk for P.A.D. complications, such as gangrene (tissue death) in the leg from decreased blood flow.

## Older Age

Older age also is a risk factor for P.A.D. Plaque builds up in your arteries as you age. Older age combined with other risk factors, such as smoking or diabetes, also puts you at higher risk for P.A.D.

## Diseases And Conditions

Many diseases and conditions can raise your risk of P.A.D., including:

- Coronary heart disease

- Diabetes

- High blood pressure

- High blood cholesterol

- Metabolic syndrome

- Stroke

# What Are The Signs And Symptoms Of Peripheral Artery Disease?

Many people who have peripheral artery disease (P.A.D.) don't have any signs or symptoms.

Even if you don't have signs or symptoms, ask your doctor whether you should get checked for P.A.D. if you're:

- Aged 70 or older

- Aged 50 or older and have a history of smoking or diabetes

- Younger than 50 and have diabetes and one or more risk factors for atherosclerosis

## Intermittent Claudication

People who have P.A.D. may have symptoms when walking or climbing stairs, which may include pain, numbness, aching, or heaviness in the leg muscles. Symptoms also may include cramping in the affected leg(s) and in the buttocks, thighs, calves, and feet. Symptoms may ease after resting. These symptoms are called intermittent claudication.

During physical activity, your muscles need increased blood flow. If your blood vessels are narrowed or blocked, your muscles won't get enough blood, which will lead to symptoms. When resting, the muscles need less blood flow, so the symptoms will go away.

## Other Signs And Symptoms

Other signs and symptoms of P.A.D. include:

- Weak or absent pulses in the legs or feet

- Sores or wounds on the toes, feet, or legs that heal slowly, poorly, or not at all

- A pale or bluish color to the skin

- A lower temperature in one leg compared to the other leg

- Poor nail growth on the toes and decreased hair growth on the legs

- Erectile dysfunction, especially among men who have diabetes

# How Is Peripheral Artery Disease Diagnosed?

Peripheral artery disease (P.A.D.) is diagnosed based on your medical and family histories, a physical exam, and test results.

P.A.D. often is diagnosed after symptoms are reported. A correct diagnosis is important because people who have P.A.D. are at higher risk for coronary heart disease (CHD), heart attack, stroke, and transient ischemic attack ("mini-stroke"). If you have P.A.D., your doctor also may want to check for signs of these diseases and conditions.

## Specialists Involved

Primary care doctors, such as internists and family doctors, may treat people who have mild P.A.D. For more advanced P.A.D., a vascular specialist may be involved. This is a doctor who specializes in treating blood vessel diseases and conditions.

A cardiologist also may be involved in treating people who have P.A.D. Cardiologists treat heart problems, such as CHD and heart attack, which often affect people who have P.A.D.

## Medical And Family Histories

Your doctor may ask:

- Whether you have any risk factors for P.A.D. For example, he or she may ask whether you smoke or have diabetes.

- About your symptoms, including any symptoms that occur when walking, exercising, sitting, standing, or climbing.

- About your diet.

- About any medicines you take, including prescription and over-the-counter medicines.

- Whether anyone in your family has a history of heart or blood vessel diseases.

## Physical Exam

During the physical exam, your doctor will look for signs of P.A.D. He or she may check the blood flow in your legs or feet to see whether you have weak or absent pulses.

Your doctor also may check the pulses in your leg arteries for an abnormal whooshing sound called a bruit. He or she can hear this sound with a stethoscope. A bruit may be a warning sign of a narrowed or blocked artery.

Your doctor may compare blood pressure between your limbs to see whether the pressure is lower in the affected limb. He or she also may check for poor wound healing or any changes in your hair, skin, or nails that may be signs of P.A.D.

## Diagnostic Tests

### Ankle-Brachial Index

A simple test called an ankle-brachial index (ABI) often is used to diagnose P.A.D. The ABI compares blood pressure in your ankle to blood pressure in your arm. This test shows how well blood is flowing in your limbs.

ABI can show whether P.A.D. is affecting your limbs, but it won't show which blood vessels are narrowed or blocked.

A normal ABI result is 1.0 or greater (with a range of 0.90 to 1.30). The test takes about 10 to 15 minutes to measure both arms and both ankles. This test may be done yearly to see whether P.A.D. is getting worse.

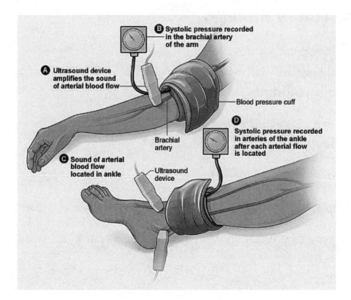

**Figure 47.2.** Ankle-Brachial Index

*The illustration shows the ankle-brachial index test. The test compares blood pressure in the ankle to blood pressure in the arm. As the blood pressure cuff deflates, the blood pressure in the arteries is recorded.*

### Doppler Ultrasound

A Doppler ultrasound looks at blood flow in the major arteries and veins in the limbs. During this test, a handheld device is placed on your body and passed back and forth over the affected area. A computer converts sound waves into a picture of blood flow in the arteries and veins.

The results of this test can show whether a blood vessel is blocked. The results also can help show the severity of P.A.D.

## Treadmill Test

A treadmill test can show the severity of symptoms and the level of exercise that brings them on. You'll walk on a treadmill for this test. This shows whether you have any problems during normal walking.

You may have an ABI test before and after the treadmill test. This will help compare blood flow in your arms and legs before and after exercise.

## Magnetic Resonance Angiogram

A magnetic resonance angiogram (MRA) uses magnetic and radio wave energy to take pictures of your blood vessels. This test is a type of magnetic resonance imaging (MRI).

An MRA can show the location and severity of a blocked blood vessel. If you have a pacemaker, man-made joint, stent, surgical clips, mechanical heart valve, or other metallic devices in your body, you might not be able to have an MRA. Ask your doctor whether an MRA is an option for you.

## Arteriogram

An arteriogram provides a "road map" of the arteries. Doctors use this test to find the exact location of a blocked artery.

For this test, dye is injected through a needle or catheter (tube) into one of your arteries. This may make you feel mildly flushed. After the dye is injected, an X-ray is taken. The X-ray can show the location, type, and extent of the blockage in the artery.

Some doctors use a newer method of arteriogram that uses tiny ultrasound cameras. These cameras take pictures of the insides of the blood vessels. This method is called intravascular ultrasound.

## Blood Tests

Your doctor may recommend blood tests to check for P.A.D. risk factors. For example, blood tests can help diagnose conditions such as diabetes and high blood cholesterol.

# How Is Peripheral Artery Disease Treated?

Treatments for peripheral artery disease (P.A.D.) include heart-healthy lifestyle changes, medicines, and surgery or procedures.

The overall goals of treating P.A.D. include reducing risk of heart attack and stroke; reducing symptoms of claudication; improving mobility and overall quality of life; and preventing complications. Treatment is based on your signs and symptoms, risk factors, and the results of physical exams and tests.

Treatment may slow or stop the progression of the disease and reduce the risk of complications. Without treatment, P.A.D. may progress, resulting in serious tissue damage in the form of sores or gangrene (tissue death) due to inadequate blood flow. In extreme cases of P.A.D., also referred to as critical limb ischemia (CLI), removal (amputation) of part of the leg or foot may be necessary.

## Heart-Healthy Lifestyle Changes

Treatment often includes making life-long heart-healthy lifestyle changes such as:

- Physical activity

- Quitting smoking

- Heart-healthy eating

## Surgery Or Procedures

### Bypass Grafting

Your doctor may recommend bypass grafting surgery if blood flow in your limb is blocked or nearly blocked. For this surgery, your doctor uses a blood vessel from another part of your body or a synthetic tube to make a graft.

This graft bypasses (that is, goes around) the blocked part of the artery. The bypass allows blood to flow around the blockage. This surgery doesn't cure P.A.D., but it may increase blood flow to the affected limb.

### Angioplasty And Stent Placement

Your doctor may recommend angioplasty to restore blood flow through a narrowed or blocked artery.

During this procedure, a catheter (thin tube) with a balloon at the tip is inserted into a blocked artery. The balloon is then inflated, which pushes plaque outward against the artery wall. This widens the artery and restores blood flow.

A stent (a small mesh tube) may be placed in the artery during angioplasty. A stent helps keep the artery open after angioplasty is done. Some stents are coated with medicine to help prevent blockages in the artery.

## Atherectomy

Atherectomy is a procedure that removes plaque buildup from an artery. During the procedure, a catheter is used to insert a small cutting device into the blocked artery. The device is used to shave or cut off plaque.

The bits of plaque are removed from the body through the catheter or washed away in the bloodstream (if they're small enough).

Doctors also can perform atherectomy using a special laser that dissolves the blockage.

## Other Types Of Treatment

Researchers are studying cell and gene therapies to treat P.A.D. However, these treatments aren't yet available outside of clinical trials.

# How Can Peripheral Artery Disease Be Prevented?

Taking action to control your risk factors can help prevent or delay peripheral artery disease (P.A.D.) and its complications. Know your family history of health problems related to P.A.D. If you or someone in your family has the disease, be sure to tell your doctor. Controlling risk factors includes the following.

- Be physically active

- Be screened for P.A.D. A simple office test, called an ankle-brachial index or ABI, can help determine whether you have P.A.D.

- Follow heart-healthy eating

- If you smoke, quit. Talk with your doctor about programs and products that can help you quit smoking.

- If you're overweight or obese, work with your doctor to create a reasonable weight-loss plan.

251

The lifestyle changes described above can reduce your risk of developing P.A.D. These changes also can help prevent and control conditions that can be associated with P.A.D., such as coronary heart disease, diabetes, high blood pressure, high blood cholesterol, and stroke.

# Chapter 48

# Sexual Health And Reproduction

## What You Should Know About Smoking And Reproduction

For many reasons, men and women who want to have children should not smoke. Studies have long shown that smoking and exposure to tobacco smoke are harmful to reproductive health. The latest Surgeon General's Report on smoking and health says that tobacco use during pregnancy remains a major preventable cause of disease and death of mother, fetus, and infant, and smoking before pregnancy can reduce fertility.

## Male Sexual Function And Fertility

Smoking is also a cause of erectile dysfunction (ED), a condition that currently affects 18 million American men over age 20. ED is defined as the inability to maintain an erection that is adequate for satisfactory sexual performance; this can affect reproduction. Cigarette smoke alters blood flow needed for an erection, and smoking interferes with the healthy function of blood vessels in erectile tissue.

About This Chapter: Text beginning with the heading "What You Should Know About Smoking And Reproduction" is excerpted from "Smoking And Reproduction," Centers for Disease Control and Prevention (CDC), October 15, 2014; Text beginning with the heading "How Does Smoking During Pregnancy Harm My Health And My Baby?" is excerpted from "Tobacco Use And Pregnancy," Centers for Disease Control and Prevention (CDC), July 20, 2016.

## Failure To Launch

Smoking increases the risk of erectile dysfunction or impotence—the inability to achieve or maintain an erection. Tar and chemicals in cigarette smoke cause damage to the blood vessels and arteries that deliver blood to the penis. Without adequate blood flow, the penis can't get or stay hard. Smoking also raises your blood pressure, which can restrict blood flow to the penis.

## Difficulty Having Kids

Toxins from cigarette smoke can damage the genetic material in sperm. Males who smoke have more damaged sperm than males who don't. Damaged sperm can cause infertility or genetic defects problems in their children. Smoking is also associated with having a low sperm count and having sperm that are "poor swimmers" which can further reduce the odds of having a child.

## Sexual Healing

If you quit smoking now, you can lower your chances of erectile dysfunction and improve your chances of having a healthy sexual life as an adult.

*(Source: "Erectile Dysfunction," Smokefree.gov, June 20, 2012.)*

# How Does Smoking During Pregnancy Harm My Health And My Baby?

Most people know that smoking causes cancer, heart disease, and other major health problems. Smoking during pregnancy causes additional health problems, including premature birth (being born too early), certain birth defects, and infant death.

- Smoking makes it harder for a woman to get pregnant.

- Women who smoke during pregnancy are more likely than other women to have a miscarriage.

- Smoking can cause problems with the placenta—the source of the baby's food and oxygen during pregnancy. For example, the placenta can separate from the womb too early, causing bleeding, which is dangerous to the mother and baby.

- Smoking during pregnancy can cause a baby to be born too early or to have low birth weight—making it more likely the baby will be sick and have to stay in the hospital longer. A few babies may even die.

- Smoking during and after pregnancy is a risk factor of Sudden Infant Death Syndrome (SIDS). SIDS is an infant death for which a cause of the death cannot be found.

- Babies born to women who smoke are more likely to have certain birth defects, like a cleft lip or cleft palate.

## What Are E-Cigarettes? Are They Safer Than Regular Cigarettes In Pregnancy?

Electronic cigarettes (also called electronic nicotine delivery systems or e-cigarettes) come in different sizes and shapes, including "pens," "mods," (i.e., these types are modified by the user) and "tanks." Most e-cigarettes contain a battery, a heating device, and a cartridge to hold liquid. The liquid typically contains nicotine, flavorings, and other chemicals. The battery-powered device heats the liquid in the cartridge into an aerosol that the user inhales.

Although the aerosol of e-cigarettes generally has fewer harmful substances than cigarette smoke, e-cigarettes and other products containing nicotine are not safe to use during pregnancy. Nicotine is a health danger for pregnant women and developing babies and can damage a developing baby's brain and lungs. Also, some of the flavorings used in e-cigarettes may be harmful to a developing baby.

## How Many Women Smoke During Pregnancy?

According to the 2011 Pregnancy Risk Assessment and Monitoring System (PRAMS) data from 24 states

- Approximately 10 percent of women reported smoking during the last 3 months of pregnancy.

- Of women who smoked 3 months before pregnancy, 55 percent quit during pregnancy. Among women who quit smoking during pregnancy, 40 percent started smoking again within 6 months after delivery.

## What Are The Benefits Of Quitting?

Quitting smoking will help you feel better and provide a healthier environment for your baby.

When you stop smoking

- Your baby will get more oxygen, even after just one day of not smoking.

- There is less risk that your baby will be born too early.

- There is a better chance that your baby will come home from the hospital with you.

- You will be less likely to develop heart disease, stroke, lung cancer, chronic lung disease, and other smoke-related diseases.

- You will be more likely to live to know your grandchildren.

- You will have more energy and breathe more easily.

- Your clothes, hair, and home will smell better.

- Your food will taste better.

- You will have more money that you can spend on other things.

- You will feel good about what you have done for yourself and your baby.

## How Does Other People's Smoke (Secondhand Smoke) Harm My Health And My Child's Health?

Breathing other people's smoke make children and adults who do not smoke sick. There is no safe level of breathing others people's smoke.

- Pregnant women who breathe other people's cigarette smoke are more likely to have a baby who weighs less.

- Babies who breathe in other people's cigarette smoke are more likely to have ear infections and more frequent asthma attacks.

- Babies who breathe in other people's cigarette smoke are more likely to die from Sudden Infant Death Syndrome (SIDS). SIDS is an infant death for which a cause of the death cannot be found.

In the United States, 58 million children and adults who do not smoke are exposed to other people's smoke. Almost 25 million children and adolescents aged 3–19 years, or about 4 out of 10 children in this age group, are exposed to other people's cigarette smoke. Home and vehicles are the places where children are most exposed to cigarette smoke, and a major location of smoke exposure for adults too. Also, people can be exposed to cigarette smoke in public places, restaurants, and at work.

# What Can You Do To Avoid Other People's Smoke?

There is no safe level of exposure to cigarette smoke. Breathing even a little smoke can be harmful. The only way to fully protect yourself and your loved ones from the dangers of other people's smoke is through 100 percent smokefree environments.

You can protect yourself and your family by

- Making your home and car smokefree.

- Asking people not to smoke around you and your children.

- Making sure that your children's day care center or school is smokefree.

- Choosing restaurants and other businesses that are smokefree. Thanking businesses for being smokefree.

- Teaching children to stay away from other people's smoke.

- Avoiding all smoke. If you or your children have respiratory conditions, if you have heart disease, or if you are pregnant, the dangers are greater for you.

- Learn as much as you can by talking to your doctor, nurse, or healthcare provider about the dangers of other people's smoke.

# Part Five
## Tobacco Use Cessation

# Chapter 49
# Ways To Quit Smoking

## Health Risks Of Smoking And Ways To Quit
### Quitting Smoking Improves Health

The risk of most health problems from smoking, including cancer and heart and lung disease, can be lowered by stopping smoking. People of all ages can improve their health if they quit smoking. Quitting at a younger age will improve a person's health even more. People who quit smoking cut their risk of lung cancer by 30 percent to 50 percent after 10 years compared to people who keep smoking, and they cut their risk of cancer of the mouth or esophagus in half within 5 years after quitting.

The damage caused by smoking is even worse for people who have had cancer. They have an increased risk of cancer recurrence, new cancers, and long-term side effects from cancer treatment. Quitting smoking and stopping other unhealthy behaviors can improve long-term health and quality of life.

The Public Health Service has a set of guidelines called Treating Tobacco Use and Dependence. It asks healthcare professionals to talk to their patients about the health problems caused by smoking and the importance of quitting smoking.

About This Chapter: Text under the heading "Health Risks Of Smoking And Ways To Quit" is excerpted from "Cigarette Smoking: Health Risks And How To Quit (PDQ®)—Patient Version," National Cancer Institute (NCI), September 8, 2016; Text under the heading "Smokefree Mobile Apps" is excerpted from "Smokefree Apps," Smokefree.gov, U.S. Department of Health and Human Services (HHS), June 3, 2015.

> ## Slips Happen
>
> Quitting smoking is a process. It may take time. During that time, you might get frustrated. There's a chance you might slip at some point and smoke a cigarette. Slips happen to a lot of people who quit smoking.
>
> (Source: "How To Support Your Quitter," Smokefree.gov, July 20, 2016.)

## Different Ways To Quit Smoking

The following are the most common methods used to help smokers quit:

### Counseling

People who have even a short counseling session with a healthcare professional are more likely to quit smoking. Your doctor or other healthcare professional may take the following steps to help you quit:

- Ask about your smoking habits at every visit

- Advise you to stop smoking

- Ask you how willing you are to quit

- Help you plan to quit smoking by:

    - setting a date to quit smoking

    - giving you self-help materials

    - recommending drug treatment

- Plan follow-up visits with you

The Lung Health Study found that heavy smokers who received counseling from a doctor, took part in group sessions with other smokers to change their behavior, and used nicotine gum were more likely to quit smoking compared with smokers who did not receive counseling from a doctor, take part in group sessions, and use nicotine gum. They also had a lower risk of lung cancer, other cancers, heart disease, and respiratory disease.

Childhood cancer survivors who smoke may be more likely to quit when they take part in programs that use peer-counseling. In these programs, childhood cancer survivors are trained in ways to give support to other childhood cancer survivors who smoke and want to quit.

More people quit smoking with peer-counseling than with self-help programs. If you are a childhood cancer survivor and you smoke, talk to your doctor about peer-counseling programs.

## Drug Treatment

Treatment with drugs is also used to help people quit smoking. These include nicotine replacement products and non-nicotine medicines. People who use any type of drug treatment are more likely to quit smoking after 6 months than those who use a placebo or no drug treatment at all.

Nicotine replacement products have nicotine in them. You slowly reduce the use of the nicotine product in order to reduce the amount of nicotine you take in. Using a nicotine replacement product can help break the addiction to nicotine. It lessens the side effects of nicotine withdrawal, such as feeling depressed or nervous, having trouble thinking clearly, or having trouble sleeping. Nicotine replacement products, used alone or in combination, have been shown to help people quit smoking. These include:

- Nicotine gum

- Nicotine patches

- Nicotine nasal spray

- Nicotine inhalers

- Nicotine lozenges

Nicotine replacement products can cause problems in some people, especially:
- Women who are pregnant or breast-feeding

- Teenagers

- People with any of the following medical problems:

  - Heart rhythm problems

  - High blood pressure that is not controlled

  - Esophagitis

  - Ulcers

  - Insulin-dependent diabetes

  - Asthma

Other medicines that do not have nicotine in them are used to help people quit smoking. These include:

- Bupropion (also called Zyban)

- Varenicline (also called Chantix)

These medicines lessen nicotine craving and nicotine withdrawal symptoms.

It is important to know that bupropion and varenicline may cause serious psychiatric problems. Symptoms include:

- Changes in behavior

- Aggressive behavior

- Anxiety

- Nervousness

- Depression

- Suicidal thoughts and attempted suicide

Varenicline may also cause serious heart problems.

Before starting to take bupropion or varenicline, talk to your doctor about the important health benefits of quitting smoking and the small but serious risk of problems with the use of these drugs.

## Smoking Reduction

When smokers do not quit smoking completely but smoke fewer cigarettes (smoking reduction) they may still benefit. The more you smoke, the higher your risk of lung cancer and other cancers related to smoking. Studies show that smokers who cut back are more likely to stop smoking in the future.

Smoking less is not as helpful as quitting smoking altogether, and is harmful if you inhale more deeply or smoke more of each cigarette to try to control nicotine cravings. In smokers who do not plan to quit smoking completely, nicotine replacement products have been shown to help them cut down the number of cigarettes they smoke, but this effect does not appear to last over time.

## Different Types Of Tobacco And Nicotine Products

The use of new or different types of tobacco products and devices that deliver nicotine is increasing rapidly in the United States, especially the use of electronic-cigarettes (e-cigarettes).

Examples of new and different tobacco and nicotine products and devices include the following:

- E-cigarettes

- Small cigars

- Water pipes (hookahs) for smoking tobacco

- Flavored smokeless tobacco products

# Smokefree Mobile Apps

Get 24/7 help with a Smokefree app for your smartphone. These free apps give you the support and skills you need to get ready to quit and stay smokefree. Explore the apps to discover the features that will be most helpful for your smokefree journey.

## QuitGuide

QuitGuide is a free app that helps you understand your smoking patterns and build the skills needed to become and stay smokefree. New to QuitGuide in 2016 is the ability to track cravings by time of day and location. Get inspirational messages for each craving you track, which keep you focused and motivated on your smokefree journey.

QuitGuide helps you:

- Track craving and slips by times of day and location

- Track your mood and smoking triggers

- Stay motivated with inspirational messages

- Identify your reasons for quitting

- Get tips and distractions for dealing with cravings and bad moods

- Monitor your progress toward achieving smokefree milestones

- Create journal entries

## quitSTART

quitSTART is a free app made for teens who want to quit smoking, but adults can use it too. This app takes the information you provide about your smoking history and gives you tailored tips, inspiration, and challenges to help you become smokefree and live a healthier life.

quitStart App helps you:

- Get ready to quit with tips and information to prepare you for becoming smokefree

- Monitor your progress and earn badges for smokefree milestones and other achievements

- Get back on track if you slip and smoke

- Manage cravings and bad moods in healthy ways

- Distract yourself from cravings with games and challenges

- Store helpful tips, inspirations, and challenges in your Quit Kit

- Share your progress and favorite tips through social media

# Chapter 50
# Preparing To Quit Smoking

Cigarette smoking harms nearly every organ of the body, causes many diseases, and reduces the health of smokers in general.

Quitting smoking lowers your risk for smoking-related diseases and can add years to your life.

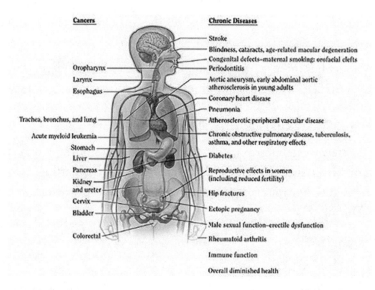

**Cancers**
- Oropharynx
- Larynx
- Esophagus
- Trachea, bronchus, and lung
- Acute myeloid leukemia
- Stomach
- Liver
- Pancreas
- Kidney and ureter
- Cervix
- Bladder
- Colorectal

**Chronic Diseases**
- Stroke
- Blindness, cataracts, age-related macular degeneration
- Congenital defects–maternal smoking: orofacial clefts
- Periodontitis
- Aortic aneurysm, early abdominal aortic atherosclerosis in young adults
- Coronary heart disease
- Pneumonia
- Atherosclerotic peripheral vascular disease
- Chronic obstructive pulmonary disease, tuberculosis, asthma, and other respiratory effects
- Diabetes
- Reproductive effects in women (including reduced fertility)
- Hip fractures
- Ectopic pregnancy
- Male sexual function–erectile dysfunction
- Rheumatoid arthritis
- Immune function
- Overall diminished health

*Figure 50.1.* Health Effects Of Smoking

About This Chapter: Text in this chapter begins with excerpts from "Health Effects Of Cigarette Smoking," Centers for Disease Control and Prevention (CDC), February 17, 2016; Text under the heading "Prepare To Quit" is excerpted from "Prepare To Quit," Smokefree.gov, U.S. Department of Health and Human Services (HHS), May 8, 2016.

# Prepare To Quit

Quitting is hard. But quitting can be a bit easier if you have a plan. When you think you're ready to quit, here are a few simple steps you can take to put your plan into action.

## Know Why You're Quitting

Before you actually quit, it's important to know why you're doing it. Do you want to be healthier? Save money? Keep your family safe? If you're not sure, ask yourself these questions:

- What do I dislike about smoking?

- What do I miss out on when I smoke?

- How is smoking affecting my health?

- What will happen to me and my family if I keep smoking?

- How will my life get better when I quit?

## Learn How To Handle Your Triggers And Cravings

Triggers are specific persons, places, or activities that make you feel like smoking. Knowing your smoking triggers can help you learn to deal with them.

Cravings are short but intense urges to smoke. They usually only last a few minutes. Plan ahead and come up with a list of short activities you can do when you get a craving.

## Find Ways To Handle Nicotine Withdrawal

During the first few weeks after you quit, you may feel uncomfortable and crave a cigarette. This is because of withdrawal. During withdrawal, your body is getting used to not having nicotine from cigarettes. For most people, the worst symptoms of withdrawal last a few days to a few weeks. During this time, you may:

- Feel a little depressed

- Be unable to sleep

- Become cranky, frustrated, or mad

- Feel anxious, nervous, or restless

- Have trouble thinking clearly

You may be tempted to smoke to relieve these feelings. Just remember that they are temporary, no matter how powerful they feel at the time.

One of the best ways to deal with nicotine withdrawal is to try nicotine replacement therapy (NRT). NRT can reduce withdrawal symptoms. And NRT can double your chances of quitting smoking for good. NRT comes in several different forms, including gum, patch, nasal spray, inhaler, and lozenge. Many are available without a prescription.

A lot of research has been done on NRT. It has been shown to be safe and effective for almost all smokers who want to quit, including teens. But if you have a severe medical condition or are pregnant, talk to your doctor about using NRT.

If you plan to use NRT, remember to have it available on your quit day. Read the instructions on the NRT package and follow them carefully. NRT will give you the most benefit if you use it as recommended.

## Explore Your Quit Smoking Options

It is difficult to quit smoking on your own, but quitting "cold turkey" is not your only choice. In fact, choosing another option may improve your chances of success. Check out:

- SmokefreeTXT text message program

- QuitGuide app

- Quitlines like 1-800-QUIT-NOW (1-800-784-8669) and 1-877-44U-QUIT (1-877-448-7848)

## Tell Your Family And Friends You Plan To Quit

Quitting smoking is easier when the people in your life support you. Let them know you are planning to quit and explain how they can help. Here are a few tips:

- Tell your family and friends your reasons for quitting.

- Ask them to check in with you to see how things are going.

- Ask them to help you think of smokefree activities you can do together (like going to the movies or a nice restaurant).

- Ask a friend or family member who smokes to quit with you, or at least not smoke around you.

- Ask your friends and family not to give you a cigarette—no matter what you say or do.

- Alert your friends and family that you may be in a bad mood while quitting. Ask them to be patient and help you through it.

## Make A Quit Plan

- Set your quit date: Start by setting your quit date. Choose a day within the next two weeks. This will give you enough time to prepare.

- Choose your reasons for quitting: Select your reasons for quitting, such as being healthier, saving money, smelling better, or for your loved ones. They will be added to your quit plan.

- Identify your smoking triggers: Knowing your emotional, habitual, or social triggers helps you stay in control. When you first quit, you might want to completely avoid your triggers. After staying smokefree for a while, you may find other ways to handle your triggers.

- Prepare to fight your cravings: Cravings only last a few minutes—but those minutes can be hard. Select the types of cravings you usually have. The tips for beating these cravings will be added to your quit plan.

- Get rid of smoking reminders: Seeing reminders of smoking makes it harder to stay smokefree. Get rid of any reminders in your home, car, and workplace before your quit day. Below is a list of common smoking reminders and how to deal with them.

- Wash your clothing, especially the jacket you wear to take smoke breaks.

- Clean your car.

- Get rid of matches, ashtrays, and any cigarette butts that may be outside your home.

- Put craving fighting items—like straws, nicotine gum, or a list of chores—in the places where you kept your cigarettes, ashtrays, matches, and lighters.

- The night before quit day, throw away everything that is related to smoking. Don't hide a pack in your freezer or stash your ashtrays in the back of a cabinet.

## Tips To Fight Cravings

1. Do you need to keep your hands and mouth busy?
   - Hold a straw in your hand and breathe through it.
   - Play with a coin or paperclip to keep your hands busy.
2. Do you smoke to relieve stress or improve your mood?
   - Practice deep breathing to calm down or do some pushups to blow off steam.

- Turn to friends, family, and counselors when you need someone to talk to.

3. Do you have trouble keeping busy and your mind occupied?

- Make a list of tasks that you can accomplish when a craving hits. This list can include chores, replying to emails, running errands, or planning your schedule for the next day.

4. Do you smoke because it's pleasurable and relaxing?

- Treat yourself to a different pleasure. Listen to your favorite songs, plan a movie night with friends, or save up your cigarette money for a special treat when you reach a smokefree milestone.

5. Do you get irritable and anxious without cigarettes?

- Nicotine replacement therapy (NRT), such as patches, gum, or lozenges, can help relieve your withdrawal symptoms. Talk to your doctor to see which type of NRT is right for you.

6. Do you smoke for an energy boost?

- To keep your energy level stable, get regular exercise and have healthy snacks throughout the day.

- Make sure you're getting plenty of sleep at night to help you from feeling slow during the day.

## EVERYTHING MUST GO!

- Tell friends and family: Quitting smoking is easier when you have support from your loved ones. Let your family and friends know that you are quitting, or invite a friend to quit with you.

Get rid of smoking reminders: Seeing reminders of smoking makes it harder to stay smoke-free. Get rid of any reminders in your home, car, and workplace before your quit day. Below is a list of common smoking reminders and how to deal with them.

# Chapter 51
# Putting A Stop To Smoky Thinking

It can be easy to lose sight of the benefits of quitting when a strong craving for a cigarette hits. You might start to lose your focus on staying smokefree. There is no good reason to smoke. You know this. So if you are giving yourself a reason to smoke, you are probably experiencing an attack of smoky thinking.

## Smoky Thinking Thoughts And Clear Thinking Responses

- **Smoky Thinking:** I just need one cigarette to take the edge off these cravings.

- **Clear Thinking:** Cravings become weaker and less frequent with every day that I don't smoke. Even just one puff will feed the cravings and make them stronger.

- **Smoky Thinking:** It's been a long day. I deserve a cigarette.

- **Clear Thinking:** I deserve a reward after a long day, but there are better rewards than a cigarette. A favorite meal, a funny movie, or a hot shower will help me relax without ruining my quit attempt.

- **Smoky Thinking:** The urge to smoke is just too strong. I can't stand it.

- **Clear Thinking:** Even the strongest cravings last less than 3 minutes. The urge will go away whether I smoke or not, and smoking now will just make it even harder for me to quit later. I can find something else to do—anything—until the craving goes away.

About This Chapter: This chapter includes text excerpted from "Putting A Stop To Smoky Thinking," Smokefree. gov, U.S. Department of Health and Human Services (HHS), November 30, 2012. Reviewed December 2016.

- **Smoky Thinking:** I blew it. I smoked a cigarette. I might as well go ahead and finish the pack.

- **Clear Thinking:** I am still learning how to be a non-smoker. It's normal to make some mistakes. But I don't have to smoke that next cigarette. I can learn from this mistake and keep going.

- **Smoky Thinking:** I can't deal with never being able to have another cigarette for the rest of my life.

- **Clear Thinking:** I only have to deal with today. Quitting happens one day at a time, sometimes one hour at a time! The future will take care of itself.

- **Smoky Thinking:** I am doing really well. Just one cigarette won't hurt.

- **Clear Thinking:** I have never smoked just one before. One cigarette always leads to another. I don't want to undo all my progress by smoking a cigarette now.

- **Smoky Thinking:** I am too grumpy without my cigarettes. I am doing my friends and family a favor by smoking.

- **Clear Thinking:** My friends and family love me and understand that quitting smoking now is the best gift I can give them. Grumpy or not, I am not doing them any favors by continuing to smoke.

- **Smoky Thinking:** I've been smoking for so long; quitting won't make a difference now.

- **Clear Thinking:** No matter how long I've been smoking, my body will benefit from quitting. The healing process starts right away, and before long I will start to feel healthier and look better.

- **Smoky Thinking:** I know people who smoked their whole lives and never got sick.

- **Clear Thinking:** It's true that some people get lucky. But there is no way of knowing whether I will be one of the lucky ones, and I am not willing to risk my life. The only safe choice is to quit smoking now.

- **Smoky Thinking:** I have already cut down to a safe level.

- **Clear Thinking:** There is no safe level of smoking. Smoking less is a good first step, but there are many more benefits when I don't smoke at all. Plus, every cigarette that I smoke feeds the habit and makes it that much harder to quit.

- **Smoky Thinking:** It's too hard to quit smoking. I can't do this.

- **Clear Thinking:** Quitting and staying away from cigarettes is hard, but it's not impossible. About 40,000,000 Americans have quit smoking. If other people can do it, so can I. It is too important to give up on.

# Chapter 52
# Smoking Cessation Products

If you want to quit smoking, you'll need willpower—and perhaps a product that's intended to help you beat the addiction.

The U.S. Food and Drug Administration (FDA) has approved a variety of smoking cessation products. These include prescription medicines as well as over-the-counter (OTC) products such as skin patches, lozenges, and gum.

Smoking cessation products are regulated through FDA's Center for Drug Evaluation and Research, which ensures that the products are safe and effective and that their benefits outweigh any known associated risks.

## First, Learn About The Products

While these products are intended to help you quit smoking and improve your health, it's important to know how they work and what side effects they may cause.

For example, many approved smoking cessation products help users wean themselves from smoking by using specific amounts of nicotine, the drug in the tobacco plant which is primarily responsible for people's addiction to tobacco products.

And, as is the case with all medications, consumers must weigh the benefits and risks as well as other considerations associated with the various products. Reading labels and talking to your pharmacist and other healthcare professionals are good initial steps to take when considering the use of smoking cessation products.

About This Chapter: Text in this chapter begins with excerpts from "FDA 101: Smoking Cessation Products," U.S. Food and Drug Administration (FDA), March 9, 2015; Text under the heading "Medications To Help You Quit Smoking" is excerpted from "Which Quit Smoking Medication Is Right For You?" Smokefree.gov, U.S. Department of Health and Human Services (HHS), July 30, 2013.

## The Benefits Of Stopping

Overcoming the addiction to smoking will bring you a multitude of benefits. According to the National Institutes of Health (NIH), not only will you lower your risk of getting various cancers, including lung cancer, you'll also reduce your chances of suffering from heart disease, stroke, emphysema, and other serious diseases. Also, quitting will help prevent heart disease and lung cancer in people who otherwise would be exposed to your second-hand smoke.

Although there are benefits to quitting at any age, it is important to quit as early in life as possible to avoid getting one of the serious illnesses caused by smoking.

Keep in mind that:

• According to the Centers for Disease Control and Prevention (CDC), more than 16 million Americans suffer from a disease caused by smoking.

• if you do not quit smoking, you have a 50 percent chance of dying of a smoking-related disease.

## Nicotine Replacement Products

Nicotine replacement is one category of smoking cessation product. Designed to wean your body off cigarettes, they supply you with nicotine in controlled amounts while sparing you from other chemicals found in tobacco products.

As you go about quitting smoking, you may experience symptoms of nicotine withdrawal. These symptoms—which include a craving, or urge, to smoke, depression, trouble sleeping, irritability, anxiety, and increased appetite—may occur no matter which method of stopping you choose.

Available over the counter and by prescription, nicotine replacement products should usually be used for a short time to help you manage nicotine cravings and withdrawal. However, FDA recognizes that some people may find that they need to use these products longer to stay smokefree. FDA has determined that there do not appear to be significant safety concerns if smokers use nicotine replacement products in combination with another product, for example, a long-acting skin patch with a short-acting gum or if they do not stop smoking completely before beginning to use such products. You may want to talk with your healthcare professional to find your best strategy to quit.

If you are under 18 years of age and want to quit smoking, you should talk to a healthcare professional about potential use of nicotine replacement therapies.

**OTC nicotine replacement products** are approved for sale to persons 18 years of age and older. These products are available under brand names and sometimes as generic products. They include:

- **Skin patches** known as transdermal nicotine patches. These patches are affixed to the skin, similar to how you would apply an adhesive bandage.

- **Chewing gum** also known as nicotine gum.

- **Lozenges** also known as nicotine lozenges. Lozenges are taken by dissolving in the mouth.

**Prescription-only nicotine replacement products** are available only under the brand name Nicotrol and are available both as a nasal spray and an oral inhaler.

**There is important advice** to consider before beginning a nicotine replacement therapy.

Women who are pregnant or breast-feeding should use these products only with approval from their healthcare professional.

Talk to your healthcare professional before using these products if you have

- diabetes, heart disease, asthma, or stomach ulcers

- had a recent heart attack

- high blood pressure that is not controlled with medicine

- a history of irregular heartbeat

- been prescribed medication to help you quit smoking

If you take prescription medication for depression or asthma, let your healthcare professional know if you are quitting smoking; your prescription dose may need to be adjusted.

Stop using a nicotine replacement product and call your healthcare professional if you experience any of the following symptoms: nausea, dizziness, weakness, vomiting, fast or irregular heartbeat, mouth problems with the lozenge or gum, or redness or swelling of the skin around the patch that does not go away.

Medications To Help You Quit Smoking

## How Do Quit Smoking Medicines Work?

When you first stop smoking, you may feel uncomfortable and will have the urge to smoke. This is due to withdrawal. Withdrawal is your body getting used to not having nicotine, the chemical in cigarettes that makes you want to keep smoking. Quit smoking medications help reduce feelings of withdrawal and cigarette cravings.

## Why Should I Use Quit Smoking Medications?

Using these medications can double your chances of quitting for good. They help reduce your cigarette cravings and withdrawal symptoms. They can also save you money. Quit smoking medications are usually used for a short amount of time. You will end up spending less to take these medications than to keep smoking.

## Which Quit Smoking Medications Are Available?

The most commonly used quit smoking medications are nicotine replacement therapy (NRT). NRT reduces withdrawal by giving you a little bit of nicotine, but not any of the other dangerous chemicals found in cigarettes. This satisfies your nicotine craving and lessens your urge to smoke. As you quit, you will use NRT with less and less nicotine. This allows your body to gradually get used to being without nicotine.

If you are unable to take NRT or it is not working for you, other quit smoking medications without nicotine are available. These medications can also help reduce withdrawal symptoms and cigarette cravings. You will need a prescription to use these medications. See your doctor or pharmacist to talk about your medication plan and to get a prescription.

Keep in mind that there is no "best" medication to help you quit, everyone is different. The medication information below provides an overview of FDA approved medications for smokers trying to quit. This may not include every medication currently available.

**Table 52.1.** Quit Smoking Medications

| Method | Availability | Description |
|--------|-------------|-------------|
| Bupropion | Prescription | Bupropion, also known as Zyban®, helps to reduce nicotine withdrawal and the urge to smoke. Bupropion can be used safely with NRT. |
| Varenicline | Prescription | Varenicline, also known as Chantix®, helps to reduce nicotine withdrawal and the urge to smoke. It also blocks the effects of nicotine from cigarettes if the user starts smoking again. |

## Thinking About Using Quit Smoking Medications?

When deciding to use quit smoking medications, keep in mind the following:

Talk with your doctor or pharmacist about using medications if you…

- Are pregnant or nursing.
- Have a serious medical condition
- Are currently using other medications
- Are under 18 years of age

Read the instructions on the package carefully and talk with your doctor or pharmacist if you have questions.

Most NRT products can be used alone or in combination. Talk with your doctor or pharmacist before taking more than one NRT product.

Medications alone can't do all the work. They can help with cravings and withdrawal, but they won't completely take away your urge to smoke. Even if you use medication to help you stop smoking, quitting may still be hard at times. Using other quit strategies with quit smoking medications gives you the best chance to quit. Quit strategies could include:

- Developing a quit plan
- Using quit programs such as SmokefreeTXT or calling a quitline.
- Exploring other quit options.

It is never too late to try quit smoking medications. No matter how long you have been smoking, your health will improve if you quit.

No matter how much you smoke, quit smoking medications can help you quit.

Your chance of becoming addicted to NRT is much lower as compared to cigarettes. There is less nicotine in NRT and it is delivered more slowly.

Using quit smoking medications doesn't mean you aren't strong enough to quit on your own. Using NRT can strengthen your resolve to quit and shows you are committed to quitting for yourself and others.

---

Fact: When used as directed, the nicotine patch can double your chances of quitting successfully.

*(Source: "Prepare To Quit," Smokefree.gov, U.S. Department of Health and Human Services (HHS), May 8, 2016.)*

---

# Chapter 53
# Nicotine Replacement Therapy

Many people use quit smoking medications to help reduce withdrawal feelings and cigarette cravings. These medications can double your chances of quitting for good.

Nicotine replacement therapy (NRT) is the most commonly used family of quit smoking medications. NRT reduces withdrawal feelings by giving you a small controlled amount of nicotine—but none of the other dangerous chemicals found in cigarettes. This small amount of nicotine helps satisfy your craving for nicotine and reduces the urge to smoke.

**Table 53.1.** NRT Types

| NRT Types | How To Get Them | How To Use Them |
| --- | --- | --- |
| Patch | Over the Counter | Place on the skin<br>Gives a small and steady amount of nicotine |
| Gum | Over the Counter | Chew to release nicotine<br>Chew until you get a tingling feeling, then place between cheek and gums |
| Lozenge | Over the Counter | Place in the mouth like hard candy<br>Releases nicotine as it slowly dissolves in the mouth |
| Inhaler | Prescription | Cartridge attached to a mouthpiece<br>Inhaling through the mouthpiece gives a specific amount of nicotine |
| Nasal Spray | Prescription | Pump bottle containing nicotine<br>Put into nose and spray |

About This Chapter: This chapter includes text excerpted from "Using Nicotine Replacement Therapy," Smokefree.gov, U.S. Department of Health and Human Services (HHS), May 28, 2016.

Doctors and other medical experts think NRT is the one of the most helpful tools smokers can use to quit. Some smokers have mild to moderate side effects. However, research shows that NRT is safe and effective. NRT can be an important part of almost every smoker's quit smoking strategy.

NRT comes in a variety of forms that are used in different ways. You can choose which forms you like best. Some NRT products work better than others for some people. Some people might prefer certain NRT products instead of others.

## Combining NRT With Other Strategies

NRT can't do all the work. It can help with withdrawal and cravings. But it won't completely take away the urge to smoke. Even if you use NRT to help you stop smoking, quitting can still be hard. Combining NRT with other strategies can improve your chances of quitting and staying quit. To give yourself the best chance for success, explore other quit methods you can combine with medication. Also think about:

- Developing a quit plan.

- Using quit programs such as SmokefreeTXT or calling a quitline.

- Using the QuitGuide app for tips and inspiration to help you be smokefree.

# Busting NRT Myths

**Myth: Nicotine replacement therapy (NRT) doesn't work.**

**Truth:** NRT works and can double a smoker's chances of quitting smoking for good.

Many smokers find NRT helpful for quitting. Every person is different. It might be worth trying NRT to see if it's right for you. Even if you tried NRT before, it might be worth trying again. NRT will help you the most if you follow directions carefully. Use enough and use it for the recommended time.

**Myth: If I use NRT, I won't have withdrawal symptoms or cravings from quitting smoking.**

**Truth:** You may still have withdrawal symptoms or cravings while using NRT. Try to be patient. Most people find withdrawal symptoms especially difficult the first week or two after quitting. Most smokers find withdrawal symptoms less intense when using NRT. If withdrawal symptoms continue a few days after you start using NRT, talk to your doctor or pharmacist about different NRT products that can help.

Follow NRT product directions carefully. Some NRT products (gum, lozenge, inhaler) work better if they are not used at the same time as high-acid drinks, such as sodas and fruit juices. It is safe to continue using NRT even if you slip and smoke one or two cigarettes. Staying on NRT increases your chances of getting back on track for quitting.

**Myth: If I use one NRT product, I can't use others.**

**Truth:** NRT products can be used safely together. For example, you might use long-acting NRT such as the patch with short-acting NRT such as a lozenge. Some people find both a long-acting patch and short-acting gum to be useful when cravings are high to handle withdrawal symptoms and fight off cravings.

**Myth: NRT is too expensive.**

**Truth:** Many states in the United States offer free NRT through their state quitlines. The North American Quitline Consortium has a quitline map to help you find free quit smoking support and other resources near you.

People eligible for Medicare or Medicaid also may be eligible for free NRT. In recent years, insurance coverage for NRT has expanded under many private insurance plans. Check your insurance plan to learn if you are eligible for coverage.

Even if NRT is not covered through your insurance or state quitline, the cost of NRT for several weeks will still be less than the cost of buying cigarettes.

**Myth: Some people should not use NRT.**

**Truth:** NRT has been available for more than 30 years. A great deal of research has been done on NRT. The research shows that NRT is safe and effective for almost all adults for quitting smoking. For most people, there is no need to talk to a doctor or healthcare provider before using NRT.

Pregnant women, teens, and people with serious health issues should talk to their doctor before using NRT. Serious health issues can include lung disease and heart problems. People with these problems still might be able to use NRT, but should talk to their doctor first.

# Chapter 54

# Dealing With The Effects Of Nicotine Withdrawal

## Understanding Nicotine Withdrawal

Nicotine is the main addictive substance in cigarettes and other forms of tobacco. Nicotine is a drug that affects many parts of your body, including your brain. Over time, your body and brain get used to having nicotine in them. About 80–90 percent of people who smoke regularly are addicted to nicotine.

When you stop smoking, your body has to get used to not having nicotine. That's withdrawal. Withdrawal can be uncomfortable. Some people say it feels like a mild case of the flu.

### You Can Prepare For Withdrawal

Withdrawal feelings usually are the strongest in the first week after quitting. Many people don't like how withdrawal feels. So some people start smoking again to feel better. The first week after quitting is when you are most at risk for a slip. It helps your quit attempt to be prepared and know what to expect so you can stay smokefree.

One way to be prepared is to use nicotine replacement therapy (NRT). NRT can be helpful for dealing with withdrawal and managing cravings. Almost all smokers can use NRT safely.

You can use NRT plus other helpful ways to be prepared for withdrawal. For example, you can sign up for SmokefreeTXT. SmokefreeTXT is a mobile text messaging service that offers

---

About This Chapter: Text under the heading "Understanding Nicotine Withdrawal" is excerpted from "Understanding Nicotine Withdrawal," Smokefree.gov, U.S. Department of Health and Human Services (HHS), May 28, 2016; Text beginning with the heading "What Are Some Of The Withdrawal Symptoms Associated With Quitting Smoking?" is excerpted from "How To Handle Withdrawal Symptoms And Triggers When You Decide To Quit Smoking," National Cancer Institute (NCI), October 29, 2010. Reviewed December 2016.

24/7 encouragement, advice, and tips to help smokers quit smoking and stay quit. It is a 6–8 week program, depending on when you set your quit date. You can receive 1 to 5 messages each day and additional quit support by texting one of the SmokefreeTXT keywords. You can start receiving messages a week before your quit date to help you prepare for withdrawal feelings.

Check out these other ways to be prepared for withdrawal:

- Call 1-800-QUIT-NOW (1-800-784-8669) 24/7 for information and tips on quitting smoking.

- Chat with a quit smoking counselor at LiveHelp (livehelp.cancer.gov). Monday through Friday, 8:00 a.m. to 11:00 p.m. Eastern time. Also in Spanish.

- Use the QuitGuide app for tips and inspiration to help you be smokefree.

# What Are Some Of The Withdrawal Symptoms Associated With Quitting Smoking?

Quitting smoking may cause short-term problems, especially for those who have smoked heavily for many years. These temporary changes can result in withdrawal symptoms.

Common withdrawal symptoms associated with quitting include the following:

- Nicotine cravings (nicotine is the substance in tobacco that causes addiction)

- Anger, frustration, and irritability

- Anxiety

- Depression

- Weight gain

Studies have shown that about half of smokers report experiencing at least four withdrawal symptoms (such as anger, anxiety, or depression) when they quit. People have reported other symptoms, including dizziness, increased dreaming, and headaches.

The good news is that there is much you can do to reduce cravings and manage common withdrawal symptoms. Even without medication, withdrawal symptoms and other problems subside over time. It may also help to know that withdrawal symptoms are usually worst during the first week after quitting. From that point on, the intensity usually drops over the first month. However, everyone is different, and some people have withdrawal symptoms for several months after quitting.

# What Are Some Of The Triggers For Smoking?

In addition to nicotine cravings, reminders in your daily life of times when you used to smoke may trigger you to smoke. Triggers are the moods, feelings, places, or things you do in your daily life that turn on your desire to smoke.

Triggers may include any of the following:

- Being around smokers.

- Starting the day.

- Feeling stressed.

- Being in a car.

- Drinking coffee or tea.

- Enjoying a meal.

- Drinking an alcoholic beverage.

- Feeling bored.

Knowing your triggers helps you stay in control because you can choose to avoid them or keep your mind distracted and busy when you cannot avoid them.

# What Can I Do About Nicotine Cravings?

As a smoker, you get used to having a certain level of nicotine in your body. You control that level by how much you smoke, how deeply you inhale the smoke, and the kind of tobacco you use. When you quit, cravings develop when your body wants nicotine. It takes time to break free from nicotine addiction. Also, when you see people smoking or are around other triggers, you may get nicotine cravings. Cravings are real. They are not just in your imagination. At the same time, your mood may change, and your heart rate and blood pressure may go up.

The urge to smoke will come and go. Cravings usually last only a very brief period of time. Cravings usually begin within an hour or two after you have your last cigarette, peak for several days, and may last several weeks. As the days pass, the cravings will get farther apart. Occasional mild cravings may last for 6 months.

Here are some tips for managing cravings:

- Remind yourself that they will pass.

- Avoid situations and activities that you used to associate with smoking.

- As a substitute for smoking, try chewing on carrots, pickles, apples, celery, sugarless gum, or hard candy. Keeping your mouth busy may stop the psychological need to smoke.

- Try this exercise: Take a deep breath through your nose and blow out slowly through your mouth. Repeat 10 times.

- Ask your doctor about nicotine replacement products or other medications.

# What Can I Do About Anger, Frustration, And Irritability?

After you quit smoking, you may feel edgy and short-tempered, and you may want to give up on tasks more quickly than usual. You may be less tolerant of others and get into more arguments.

Studies have found that the most common negative feelings associated with quitting are feelings of anger, frustration, and irritability. These negative feelings peak within 1 week of quitting and may last 2 to 4 weeks.

Here are some tips for managing these negative feelings:

- Remind yourself that these feelings are temporary.

- Engage in a physical activity, such as taking a walk.

- Reduce caffeine by limiting or avoiding coffee, soda, and tea.

- Try meditation or other relaxation techniques, such as getting a massage, soaking in a hot bath, or breathing deeply through your nose and out through your mouth for 10 breaths.

- Ask your doctor about nicotine replacement products or other medications.

# What Can I Do About Anxiety?

Within 24 hours of quitting smoking, you may feel tense and agitated. You may feel a tightness in your muscles—especially around the neck and shoulders. Studies have found that anxiety is one of the most common negative feelings associated with quitting. If anxiety occurs, it builds over the first 3 days after quitting and may last 2 weeks.

Here are some tips for managing anxiety:

- Remind yourself that anxiety will pass with time.

- Set aside some quiet time every morning and evening—a time when you can be alone in a quiet environment.

- Engage in physical activity, such as taking a walk.

- Reduce caffeine by limiting or avoiding coffee, soda, and tea.

- Try meditation or other relaxation techniques, such as getting a massage, soaking in a hot bath, or breathing deeply through your nose and out through your mouth for 10 breaths.

- Ask your doctor about nicotine replacement products or other medications.

# What Can I Do About Depression?

It is normal to feel sad for a period of time after you first quit smoking. If mild depression occurs, it will usually begin within the first day, continue for the first couple of weeks, and go away within a month.

Having a history of depression is associated with more severe withdrawal symptoms—including more severe depression. Some studies have found that many people with a history of major depression will have a new major depressive episode after quitting. However, in those with no history of depression, major depression after quitting is rare.

Many people have a strong urge to smoke when they feel depressed. Here are some tips for managing depression:

- Call a friend and plan to have lunch or go to a movie, concert, or other pleasurable event.

- Identify your specific feelings at the time that you seem depressed. Are you actually feeling tired, lonely, bored, or hungry? Focus on and address these specific needs.

- Increase physical activity. This will help to improve your mood and lift your depression.

- Breathe deeply.

- Make a list of things that are upsetting to you and write down solutions for them.

- If depression continues for more than 1 month, see your doctor. Ask your doctor about prescription medications that may help you with depression. Studies show that bupropion and nortriptyline can help people with a past history of depression who try to quit smoking. Nicotine replacement products also help.

# What Can I Do About Weight Gain?

Gaining weight is common after quitting. Studies have shown that, on average, people who have never smoked weigh a few pounds more than smokers, and, when smokers quit, they attain the weight they would have had if they had never smoked.

Although most smokers gain fewer than 10 pounds after they quit smoking, the weight gain can be troublesome for some people. However, the health benefits of quitting far outweigh the health risks of a small amount of extra weight.

Here are some tips for managing weight gain:

- Ask your doctor about the medication bupropion. Studies show that it helps counter weight gain.

- Studies also show that nicotine replacement products, especially nicotine gum and lozenges, can help counter weight gain. Because some people who quit smoking increase their food intake, regular physical activity and healthy food choices can help you maintain a healthy weight.

- If weight gain is a problem, you may want to consult a nutritionist or diet counselor.

# How Can I Resist The Urge To Smoke When I'm Around Smokers?

You may want to analyze situations in which watching others smoke triggers an urge in you to smoke. Figure out what it is about those situations that makes you want to smoke. Is it because you associate feeling happy with being around other smokers? Or, is there something special about the situations, such as being around the people you usually smoked with? Is it tempting to join others for routine smoke breaks?

Here are some tips:

- Limit your contact with smokers, especially in the early weeks of quitting.

- Do not buy, carry, light, or hold cigarettes for others.

- If you are in a group and others light up, excuse yourself, and don't return until they have finished.

- Do not let people smoke in your home. Post a small "No Smoking" sign by your front door.

- Ask others to help you stay quit. Give them specific examples of things that are helpful (such as not smoking around you) and things that are not helpful (like asking you to buy cigarettes for them).

- Focus on what you've gained by quitting. For example, think of how healthy you will be when all smoking effects are gone from your body and you can call yourself smokefree. Also, add up how much money you have saved already by not purchasing cigarettes and imagine (in detail) how you will spend your savings in 6 months.

## How Can I Start The Day Without Smoking?

Many smokers light up a cigarette right after they wake up. After 6 to 8 hours of sleep, a smoker's nicotine level drops and the smoker needs a boost of nicotine to start the day. After you quit, you must be ready to overcome the physical need and routine of waking up and smoking a cigarette. Instead of reaching for your cigarettes in the morning, here are some tips:

- The morning can set the tone for the rest of the day. Plan a different wake-up routine, and divert your attention from smoking.

- Be sure no cigarettes are available.

- Before you go to sleep, make a list of things you need to avoid in the morning that will make you want to smoke. Place this list where you used to place your cigarettes.

- Begin each day with a planned activity that will keep you busy for an hour or more. It will keep your mind and body busy so you don't think about smoking.

- Begin each day with deep breathing and by drinking one or more glasses of water.

## How Can I Resist The Urge To Smoke When I'm Feeling Stressed?

Most smokers report that one reason they smoke is to handle stress. This happens because smoking cigarettes actually relieves some of your stress by releasing powerful chemicals in your brain. Temporary changes in brain chemistry cause you to experience decreased anxiety, enhanced pleasure, and alert relaxation. Once you stop smoking, you may become more aware of stress.

Everyday worries, responsibilities, and hassles can all contribute to stress. As you go longer without smoking, you will get better at handling stress, especially if you learn stress reduction and relaxation techniques.

Here are some tips:

- Know the causes of stress in your life (your job, traffic, your children, money) and identify the stress signals (headaches, nervousness, or trouble sleeping). Once you pinpoint high-risk trigger situations, you can start to develop new ways to handle them.

- Create peaceful times in your everyday schedule. For example, set aside an hour where you can get away from other people and your usual environment.

- Try relaxation techniques, such as progressive relaxation or yoga, and stick with the one that works best for you.

- Rehearse and visualize your relaxation plan. Put your plan into action. Change your plan as needed.

- You may find it helpful to read a book about how to handle stress.

## How Can I Resist The Urge To Smoke When I'm Driving Or Riding In A Car?

You may have become used to smoking while driving—to relax in a traffic jam or to stay alert on a long drive. Like many smokers, you may like to light up when driving to and from work to relieve stress, stay alert, relax, or just pass the time. There is some evidence that smoking actually does make you feel more awake and alert.

Tips for short trips:

- Remove the ashtray, lighter, and cigarettes from your car.

- Keep nonfattening snacks in your car (such as licorice, sugarless gum, and hard candy).

- Turn on your favorite music and sing along.

- Take an alternate route to work or try carpooling.

- Clean your car and make sure to use deodorizers to reduce the tobacco smell.

- Tell yourself:

  - "This urge will go away in a few minutes."

  - "So, I'm not enjoying this car ride. Big deal! It won't last forever!"

  - "My car smells clean and fresh!"

  - "I'm a better driver now that I'm not smoking while driving."

When you are driving or riding with other people:

- Ask passengers not to smoke in your car.

- If you're not driving, find something to do with your hands.

Your desire to smoke may be stronger and more frequent on longer trips. Tips for long trips:

- Take a stretch break.

- Take fresh fruit along.

- Plan rest stops.

- Plan stops for water or fruit juice.

# How Can I Resist The Urge To Smoke When I'm Having Coffee Or Tea?

You may be used to smoking when drinking coffee or tea (for example, during or after meals or during work breaks), and you may associate good feelings with drinking a hot beverage. When you give up smoking, expect to feel a strong urge to reach for a cigarette while drinking coffee or tea. Although you do not have to give up coffee or tea to quit smoking, you should expect that coffee or tea will not taste the same without a cigarette.

Here are some tips:

- If you used to smoke while drinking coffee or tea, tell people you have quit, so they won't offer you a cigarette.

- Between sips of coffee or tea, take deep breaths to inhale the aroma. Breathe in deeply and slowly while you count to five, and then breathe out slowly, counting to five again.

- Try switching to decaffeinated coffee or tea for a while, particularly if quitting has made you irritable or nervous.

- Keep your hands busy by nibbling on healthy foods, doodling, or making a list of tasks for the day.

- If the urge to smoke is very strong, drink your coffee or tea more quickly than usual and then change activities or rooms.

- When you quit smoking, drinking coffee or tea without smoking may make you feel sad. Focus on what you've gained by quitting.

# How Can I Enjoy A Meal Without Smoking?

Food often tastes better after you quit smoking, and you may have a bigger appetite. Expect to want to smoke after meals. Your desire to smoke after meals may depend on whether you are alone, with other smokers, or with nonsmokers.

Your urge to smoke may be stronger with certain foods, such as spicy or sweet foods. Also, the urge to smoke may be stronger at different meal times.

Here are some tips:

- Know what kinds of foods increase your urge to smoke and stay away from them.

- If you are alone, call a friend or take a walk as soon as you've finished eating.

- Brush your teeth or use mouthwash right after meals.

- If you have coffee or a fruit drink, concentrate on the taste.

- Wash the dishes by hand after eating—you can't smoke with wet hands!

- Eat at smokefree restaurants.

# How Can I Resist The Urge To Smoke When I'm Drinking An Alcoholic Beverage?

You may be used to smoking when drinking beer, wine, liquor, or mixed drinks, and you may associate good feelings with drinking alcoholic beverages. When you quit smoking, you may feel a strong urge to smoke when you drink alcohol. Know this up front if you are going to drink. If you do drink, keep in mind that your control over your behavior may be impaired under the influence of alcohol. When you try to quit smoking, drinking alcohol may make it even tougher to cope.

Here are some tips for the first few weeks after quitting:

- Many people find it helpful to reduce or avoid drinking alcohol.

- Switch to nonalcoholic drinks.

- If you do drink, don't choose the alcoholic beverages you usually have when smoking.

- Don't drink at home or by yourself.

- Stay away from the places you usually drink alcohol, or drink only with nonsmoking friends.

# How Can I Resist The Urge To Smoke When I'm Feeling Bored?

When you quit smoking, you may miss the increased excitement and good feeling that nicotine gave you. This may be particularly true when you are feeling bored.

Here are some tips:

- Plan more activities than you have time for.

- Make a list of things to do when confronted with free time.

- Move! Do not stay in the same place too long.

- If you feel very bored when waiting for something or someone (a bus, your friend, your kids), distract yourself with a book, magazine, or crossword puzzle.

- Look at and listen to what is going on around you.

- Carry something to keep your hands busy.

- Listen to a favorite song.

- Go outdoors, if you can, but not to places you associate with smoking.

# Do Nicotine Replacement Products Relieve Nicotine Cravings And Withdrawal Symptoms?

Yes. Nicotine replacement products deliver measured doses of nicotine into the body, which helps to relieve the cravings and withdrawal symptoms often felt by people trying to quit smoking. Nicotine replacement products are effective treatments that can increase the likelihood that someone will quit successfully.

# Are Nicotine Replacement Products Safe?

It is far less harmful for a person to get nicotine from a nicotine replacement product than from cigarettes because tobacco smoke contains many toxic and cancer-causing substances. Long-term use of nicotine replacement products has not been associated with any serious harmful effects.

# Are There Alternative Methods To Help People Quit Smoking?

Some people claim that alternative approaches such as hypnosis, acupuncture, acupressure, laser therapy (laser stimulation of acupuncture points on the body), or electrostimulation may help reduce the symptoms associated with nicotine withdrawal. However, in clinical studies these alternative therapies have not been found to help people quit smoking. There is no evidence that alternative approaches help smokers who are trying to quit.

# Chapter 55

# Smokeless Tobacco: A Guide For Quitting

So you're a dipper and you'd like to quit. Maybe you've already found that quitting dip or chew is not easy. But you can do it! This chapter is intended to help you make your own plan for quitting.

Many former dippers have shared advice on quitting that can help you. Among them are many Major League Baseball players who quit successfully. This guide is the result of advice from chewers and dippers who have canned the habit.

Like most dippers, you probably know that the health-related reasons to quit are awesome. But you must find your own personal reasons for quitting. They can motivate you more than the fear of health consequences. It's important to develop your own recipe for willpower.

## The Dangers Of Dip And Chew

Here's a brief summary of the harm dipping does in the mouth:

- Spit tobacco use may cause cancer of the mouth.

- Sugar in spit tobacco may cause decay in exposed tooth roots.

- Dip and chew can cause your gums to pull away from the teeth in the place where the tobacco is held. The gums do not grow back.

- Leathery white patches and red sores are common in dippers and chewers and can turn into cancer.

About This Chapter: This chapter includes text excerpted from "Smokeless Tobacco A Guide For Quitting," National Institute of Dental and Craniofacial Research (NIDCR), August 2012. Reviewed December 2016.

# Spit Tobacco Use Can Cause Problems In Other Parts Of The Body

Recent research shows that spit tobacco use might also cause problems beyond the mouth. Some studies have shown that using spit tobacco may cause pancreatic cancer. And scientists are also looking at the possibility that its use might play a role in the development of cardio-vascular disease—heart disease and stroke.

# Need More Reasons To Quit?

## It's Expensive

A can of dip costs an average of nearly $3. A two-can-a-week habit costs about $300 per year. A can-a-day habit costs nearly $1,100 per year. Likewise, chewing tobacco costs about $2. A pouch-a-day habit costs over $700 a year. Think of all the things you could do with that money instead of dipping or chewing. It adds up.

## It's Disgusting!

If the health effects don't worry you, think of how other people see your addiction. The smell of spit tobacco in your mouth is not pleasant. While you may have become used to the odor and don't mind it, others around you notice.

Check out your clothes. Do you have tobacco juice stains on your clothes, your furniture, or on your car's upholstery?

Look at your teeth. Are they stained from tobacco juice? Brushing your teeth won't make this go away.

# Understanding Your Addiction

Nicotine, found in all tobacco products, is a highly addictive drug that acts in the brain and throughout the body.

## How Addicted Are You?

- Do you no longer get sick or dizzy when I dip or chew, like I did when I first started.

- Do you dip more often and in different settings.

- Have switched to stronger products, with more nicotine.

- Do you swallow juice from my tobacco on a regular basis.

- Do you sometimes sleep with dip or chew in my mouth.

- Do you take my first dip or chew first thing in the morning.

- Do you find it hard to go more than a few hours without dip or chew.

- Do you have strong cravings when I go without dip or chew.

## Myths And Truths

There are several myths about spit tobacco. Sometimes these myths make users feel more comfortable in their habits. Here are some myths and the truths that relate to them.

- **Myth:** Spit tobacco is a harmless alternative to smoking.
- **Truth:** Spit tobacco is still tobacco. In tobacco are nitrosamines, cancer-causing chemicals from the curing process. Note the warnings on the cans.
- **Myth:** Dip (or chew) improves my athletic performance.
- **Truth:** A study of professional baseball players found no connection between spit tobacco use and player performance. Using spit tobacco increases your heart rate and blood pressure within a few minutes. This can cause a buzz or rush, but the rise in pulse and blood pressure places an extra stress on your heart.
- **Myth:** Good gum care can offset the harmful effects of using dip or chew.
- **Truth:** There is no evidence that brushing and flossing will undo the harm that dip and chew are doing to your teeth and gums.
- **Myth:** It's easy to quit using dip or chew when you want to.
- **Truth:** Unfortunately, nicotine addiction makes quitting difficult. But those who have quit successfully are very glad they did.

# Quitting Plan

Kicking the dip or chew habit can be tough, but it can be done, and you can do it. The best way to quit spit tobacco is to have a quit date and a quitting plan. These methods make it easier. Try what you think will work best for you.

## Decide To Quit

Quitting spit tobacco is not something you do on a whim. You have to want to quit to make it through those first few weeks off tobacco. Know your reasons for stopping. Don't let outside influence—like peer pressure—get in your way. Focus on all you don't like about dipping or chewing.

## Reasons To Quit

Here are some reasons given by others. Are any of them important to you?

- To avoid health problems

- To prove I can do it

- I have sores or white patches in my mouth

- To please someone I care about

- To set a good example for my kids or other kids

- To save money

- I don't like the taste

- I have gum or tooth problems

- It's disgusting

- Because it's banned at work or school

- I don't want it to control me

- My girlfriend (or a girl I'd like to date) hates it

- My wife hates it

- My physician or dentist told me to quit

## Pick A Quit Date

Pick your quit date. Even if you think you're ready to quit now, take at least a week to get ready. But don't put off setting the date.

## Get Psyched Up For Quitting

Cut back before you quit by tapering down. Have your physician or dentist check your mouth. Ask whether you need nicotine replacement therapy (gum, nicotine patches, etc.). There is no "ideal" time to quit, but low-stress times are best. Having a quit date in mind is important, no matter how far off it is. But it's best to pick a date in the next two weeks, so you don't put it off too long.

## Cut Back Before You Quit

Some people are able to quit spit tobacco "cold turkey." Others find that cutting back makes quitting easier. There are many ways to cut back. Taper down. Cut back to half of your usual amount before you quit. If you usually carry your tin or pouch with you, try leaving it behind. Carry substitutes instead—sugar-free chewing gum or hard candies, and sunflower seeds. During this period, you might also try a mint-leaf snuff.

Cut back on when and where you dip or chew. First, notice when your cravings are strongest. What events trigger dipping or chewing for you? Do you always reach for a dip after meals? When you work out? In your car or truck? On your job? Don't carry your pouch or tin. Use a substitute instead. Go as long as you possibly can without giving into a craving—at least 10 minutes. Try to go longer and longer as you approach your quit day. Now, pick three of your strongest triggers and stop dipping or chewing at those times. This will be hard at first. The day will come when you are used to going without tobacco at the times you want it most.

Notice what friends and coworkers who don't dip or chew are doing at these times. This will give you ideas for dip or chew substitutes. It's a good idea to avoid your dipping and chewing pals while you're trying to quit. That will help you avoid the urge to reach for a can or chew.

Switch to a lower nicotine tobacco product if you're using a medium or high nicotine snuff product. This way, you cut down your nicotine dose while you're getting ready to quit. This can help to prevent strong withdrawal when you quit.

Don't switch to other tobacco products like cigarettes or cigars! In fact, if you already smoke, this is a good time to quit smoking. That way you can get over all your nicotine addiction at once.

## Build A Support Team

Let friends, family, and coworkers know you're quitting. Warn them that you may not be your usual self for a week or two after you quit. Ask them to be patient. Ask them to stand by to listen and encourage you when the going gets rough.

Suggest ways they can help, like joining you for a run or a walk, helping you find ways to keep busy, and telling you they know you can do it. If they've quit, ask them for tips. If they use dip or chew, ask them not to offer you any. They don't have to quit themselves to be supportive, but maybe someone will want to quit with you.

## Quit Day

Make your quit day special right from the beginning. You're doing yourself a huge favor.

Change daily routines to break away from tobacco triggers. When you eat breakfast, don't sit in the usual place at the kitchen table. Get right up from the table after meals. Make an appointment to get your teeth cleaned. You'll enjoy the fresh, clean feeling and a whiter smile.

Keep busy and active. Start the day with a walk, run, swim, or workout. Aerobic exercise will help you relax. Plus, it boosts energy, stamina, and all-around fitness and curbs your appetite.

Chew substitutes. Try sugar-free hard candies or gum, cinnamon sticks, mints, beef jerky, or sunflower seeds. Carry them with you and use them whenever you have the urge to dip or chew.

## Be Prepared For Temptation

Tobacco thoughts and urges probably still bother you. They will be strongest in the places where you dipped or chewed the most. The more time you spend in these places without dipping or chewing, the weaker the urges will become. Avoid alcoholic beverages. Drinking them could bust your plan to quit. Know what events and places will be triggers for you and plan ahead for them.

Write down some of your triggers. And write what you'll do instead of dip or chew. It may be as simple as reaching for gum or seeds, walking away, or thinking about how far you've come.

## Tips For Going The Distance

Congratulations! You've broken free of a tough addiction. If you can stay off 2 weeks, then you know you can beat this addiction. It will get easier.

Keep using whatever worked when you first quit. Don't expect new rituals to take the place of spit tobacco right away. It took time to get used to chewing or dipping at first, too.

Keep up your guard. Continue to plan ahead for situations that may tempt you.

## Celebrate Your Success

Congratulations! You've done it. You've beaten the spit tobacco habit. You're improving your health and your future. Celebrate with the people on your "support team." Offer your support to friends and coworkers who are trying to quit using tobacco. Pledge to yourself never to take another dip or chew.

## What If You Should Slip?

Try not to slip, not even once. But, if you do slip, get right back on track.

Don't let feelings of guilt lead you back to chewing or dipping. A slip does not mean "failure." Figure out why you slipped and how to avoid it next time. Get rid of any leftover tobacco.

# Chapter 56

# Adapting Your Social Life When Trying To Quit Smoking

You're a teenager, and your social life is important to you. But have you ever thought about how it can influence your decisions? 90 percent of adult smokers started smoking in their teens. Does who you hang out with affect your smoking? Learn more about things you can do to still have a life while you're trying to quit smoking.

## Friends

You hang out with people you have stuff in common with, right? Well, teens who smoke usually hang out with people who smoke too. So what do you do when you want to quit smoking and your friends don't? Will these relationships change while you're trying to quit smoking? It's important to know that quitting smoking could cause changes (some good and some bad) in some of your relationships and how to be ready for those changes so you can deal with them.

**Here are some things to think about:**

- **You have plenty in common:** You won't lose your friends just because you don't smoke. You and your friends have plenty of other things in common besides smoking. Remind yourself of what they are.

- **Agree to disagree:** You have your reasons for cutting back. You need to do what's right for you, but don't judge your friends who aren't ready to take the step to quit. They need to do it on their own time.

About This Chapter: This chapter includes text excerpted from "Social Life," Smokefree.gov, U.S. Department of Health and Human Services (HHS), February 15, 2012. Reviewed December 2016.

- **Who's pressuring you to smoke—you or your friends?** Most teens pressure themselves into smoking as a way to be accepted by friends. Most of your friends don't care if you say no.

- **Everyone is NOT doing it:** Most people way over estimate the number of people who are current smokers. About 80 percent of teens do NOT smoke! The tobacco companies spend a lot of money to make people think smoking is popular.

**Here are some things to do:**

- **Change up your routines and patterns:** You have routines and patterns for how you interact with and relate to other people. And you probably have patterns for smoking. Think about it. Chances are good that you smoke with the same people, at the same time, in the same place, and while you're doing the same thing (like sharing cigarettes after school or smoking in the car with your sister). You may not realize these patterns at first, but you'll need to identify them so you can begin to make changes. Mix up your routine by suggesting non-smoking activities or seeking out the company of friends who don't smoke.

- **Avoid certain social situations:** At first, it may be best to avoid social situations that trigger you to smoke. If your plan to quit involves some major changes, try explaining to your friends (and family) that you're not avoiding them, but you are avoiding situations that might make you want to smoke.

- **Ask for help: Asking for help doesn't have to be hard.** It's important to tell the people you're close to about your plan to quit. Let them know how they can help you! It can strengthen your relationships.

# Relationships

Do you remember your first time—with cigarettes, that is? Was it love at first puff? Or did you have a one night smoke and then call it quits? How about now? Still flirting? Maybe you hook up every once in awhile after school or at parties on the weekends. Or maybe you and cigarettes have started seeing a lot of each other. Could you be dating? Do you officially have a cig-nificant other?

## Not Sure What Your Relationship Status Is?

### One Night Smoke

You hit it and quit it. You tried it out, realized you didn't like smoking so you moved on.

**What this means:** You dodged a bullet. Many teens who experiment with smoking go on to become lifelong smokers—and suffer the serious health consequences. Nowadays, you are all about healthy relationships, so you won't be tempted to flirt with smoking again.

## Flings

You and cigarettes occasionally hook up at certain places or in certain situations, like parties or at a friend's house. You're experimenting with different brands and just having fun playing the field.

**What this means:** Flings can be fun, but someone usually wants to get serious after a while. Even if you only hook up once in awhile, you can get hooked—on nicotine. You may not be looking for a long-term relationship, but you should know that every time you hook up with cigarettes, you're falling farther and farther in "love."

## Friends With Benefits

You hook up with cigarettes when you're feeling stressed out. It's no strings attached, just stress relief.

**What this means:** Friends with benefits might seem like a good idea, but let's face it—somebody always gets hurt. Smoking may make you feel better temporarily, but there is no such thing as a safe cigarette. This friend with "benefits" will leave you totally damaged.

## Bromance

Cigarettes are like your wing man or wing woman. You always bring them with you wherever you go to help break the ice in new or awkward situations to get the party started.

**What this means:** Think your bro has your back? Think again. Relying on cigarettes to make you look good can backfire. Smokers are often seen as less attractive and more nervous than non-smokers. Awkward!

## Dating

You and cigarettes get together pretty regularly. You hang out every day before and after school and on the weekends. At this point in the game, you're only with one brand of cigarettes and seeing where things go.

**What this means:** Now that you and your cigarettes are spending more time together, you may start to notice some "red flags"—things that spell trouble for happily ever after. The stank that clings to your clothes and fingers after every date. The zits that won't go away. The unfortunate breath. It can be tempting to ignore these warning signs, but if you are honest with yourself you will know it's time to move on—this is not "The One."

## Facebook Official

It's official, you're in a committed relationship. You've been smoking regularly now for more than a year and you hang out pretty much 24/7. You and your cig-nificant other are going strong, and you don't have any plans to quit this relationship any time soon.

**What this means:** You are caught in a bad romance. You know the ugly, and you know the disease—but you've made a choice to stick by your cigarettes. Or maybe you are just staying because it's easier than breaking up. Whatever your reasons, remember that you do have a choice in the matter. Just because you are Facebook official doesn't mean that you can't change your mind.

No matter what your relationship status is, it's important to decide if this is what you really want. Are you in it for the long haul? You should know that the longer you stay in this relationship, the harder it will be to bail.

## Before Things Go Any Further, Ask Yourself The Following Questions About Your Relationship

### Are You Falling Harder Than You Think?

You aren't looking for a serious relationship, and you can take or leave cigarettes. At least that's what you tell yourself. But lately, you spend a lot of time thinking about cigarettes—when you will see them next, how you can get them, and the things you two might do together. You are hooking up more and more often, and you find yourself missing them when they aren't around. The truth is, you need cigarettes more than you care to admit. You don't have to smoke every day, or even every week, to get hooked on nicotine. Think about it—there's a reason you keep coming back for more.

### Is Your Relationship High Maintenance?

Do your cigarettes dictate where you go, what you do, and who you do it with? Your parents hate cigarettes, so forget about smoking at home. Cigarettes aren't allowed on school property, so you can only see each other in the parking lot after class. You can't take them to the movies, out to eat, or anywhere else normal couples go. Even worse, you have to worry about washing your hands; covering up their smell; burning other people, your car, or your clothes; and being in love with a liar.

Not only is it hard to find time for the two of you to be together, but your dates aren't exactly cheap either! Cigarettes need lighters, matches, etc., to light the fire between the two of you. Not only that, but cigarettes usually travel in packs. Smoking a pack a day can cost you about $3,000 a year!

It can be exhausting and expensive trying to keep up with the demands your partner requires! Is this relationship really worth it?

## Are You In A Toxic Relationship?

We all have that friend who's in a relationship with someone they know isn't good for them. No matter how much that person hurts them, they give it one more chance, and another, and another. Every time they get burned, they swear it's the last time and that they're not going back. But, they always do. You've seen your friends do this a hundred times, and you swore to yourself that you would never do that!

Or would you? How many chances are you willing to give cigarettes? 5? 10? 100? Every time you smoke, cigarettes are causing permanent damage to your body. Besides putting toxic chemicals into your body, cigarettes can stunt the development of your vital organs. Teens who smoke have smaller, weaker lungs than teens who don't, and may never reach their maximum lung capacity as adults. Teens who smoke also show signs of heart stress, including physical changes to the heart muscle itself, and a higher resting heart rate. These are warning signs that the heart is working extra hard. Maybe you've noticed other negative consequences from smoking too. You can't taste things when you go out to eat, you're constantly breaking out, you're always sick, your fingers and teeth are turning yellow, and you can't really see in the dark as well.

## Does Your Wingman Really Have Your Back?

Don't know what to say to the hottie you've been eyeing at the party? "No problem," you think to yourself, "I'll break the ice by asking her to bum a lighter." Want some one-on-one time with her? You just ask her to join you outside for a smoke. Your wingman's always there to help you out with the ladies.

What your wingman might not know is that about 80 percent of teens don't smoke. So breaking the ice by asking for a lighter might be a little harder than you think. Your wingman also might not know that smokers are often seen as less attractive and more nervous than non-smokers.

## Are You Staying In This Relationship Because It's Comfortable?

At this point in your relationship, you might be smoking with the same people, at the same time, in the same place, and while you're doing the same thing. Perhaps you've thought about breaking up once or twice, but you're afraid that if you do, all of your friends will hang out with your "ex" and not you. Or you'll have to find new places to hang out because of your "ex."

Have you ever thought that smoking might be holding you back from doing the things you really want to do? You'll never know unless you try! Letting go of the familiar can be scary, but you are young and have your whole life ahead of you. Do you really want to settle? Just cause you started dating doesn't mean you have to keep going—you made a choice, and you could make a different choice.

Do you know a deal breaker when you see one? Sometimes relationships, no matter how much you want to make them work or how long you've been together, just aren't good for you. It might be time to think about calling it quits. Breaking up is hard to do, but in these situations, it might be the right thing for you.

## How To Break Up With Cigarettes

When You're Ready To Call It Quits, START By Doing The Following:

- Pick a day to break up.

- Write a break up letter. It might sound dumb, but Colin Farrell wrote a break up letter to his cigarettes when he quit smoking. It's a great way to address all the reasons why your relationship isn't working anymore and help you move on.

- Figure out how you want to break up. There are many different options so check out the following to see which is right for you:

  - Breaking up via text message

  - Breaking up over the phone

  - Breaking up online

- Avoid places and situations where you and your cigarettes used to hang out. Going to these places will only remind you of your time together and may make you miss them.

- Get rid of all of the things that remind you of your "ex." Matches, lighters, ashtrays, pictures of the two of you—everything!

## Need Break Up Survival Skills?

Feeling down or stressed out about your break up? Tempted to hook back up with your "ex"? Don't do it! Whatever reasons you had for breaking up will still be there, and you'll only feel worse about your decision to hook up afterward.

# Parties

You're at a party. It's ok, but there's a part of you that isn't really sure about being there. Maybe you're bored. You feel like a cigarette would be good right about now.

It could be lots of things. Consider this: Cigarettes have been advertised as:

- A way to participate in group activities, like parties

- A way to make new friends

- A way to relieve stress

- A way to have fun

- A way to be cool and popular

Whether you're the life of the party or you're shy, cigarettes promise to make the whole night better, right? Movies tell you this. TV tells you this. Your favorite bands probably tell you this. But do you really need cigarettes to do these things?

Because you know you don't need cigarettes to do any of these things, try leaving them behind this weekend.

> Less than one in five teens smoke, so staying at the party—instead of leaving to smoke—could help you make new friends.

Those who leave the party to smoke are missing out and are often seen as less attractive and more nervous. Is that really what you want people saying about you Monday morning at school?

# Support

Get by with a little help from your friends. Life is full of ups and downs. Don't ride it out alone. Research shows that people who have close friends and family they can count on are happier and healthier. So, call on yours during the good times and the bad times. Isn't that what true friends and family are for?

**Follow these 12 tips to get the support you need:**

**1. Surround yourself with people you trust**

Think of the people you trust the most—people you can talk to about anything and who have been there for you when you needed them. Friends, parents, grandparents, teachers... whoever they are, spend more time with them.

**Tip:** Turn your everyday events into +1 activities. Grab lunch with a friend, hang out at the mall, or meet up for your school's basketball game.

## 2. Go with your gut

People change. Sometimes that means friends grow apart. Go with your gut if a friendship doesn't feel right anymore. Letting go can be hard, but you can't fly if you let people weigh you down.

**Tip:** Don't be afraid to try a little distance with people who aren't giving you the support you need. Focus your energy on spending time with people who make you feel good about yourself and want you to succeed.

## 3. Make time

Good friendships don't happen overnight. Make a point to invest time in yours. When people know your friendship is more than just a convenience for you, they'll be more willing to help you out. You'll feel more comfortable calling on them for support, too.

**Tip:** Go to that movie your friend really wants to see, even if it's not your top pick. Or go out of your way to walk a friend home after school, just so you can keep talking.

## 4. Ask for help

You might like to solve problems on your own, but the truth is we all need a little help from time to time. Go ahead and ask the people you trust. Seriously. It doesn't mean you're weak. Your true friends will be there, ready and willing to help.

**Tip:** Not sure how to ask? Send a text or IM to get the conversation started (like, I want to quit smoking. Can you help me?). Know an ex-smoker? Ask them why and how they quit.

## 5. Leave mind reading to the psychics

Unless your friends can read minds, it's safe to say they don't always know what you're thinking. Be specific about what support you want (and don't want). But be nice about it. Giving lectures is a job best left to your teachers.

**Tip:** Feeling stressed after a breakup and craving a cigarette? Tell a friend and ask them to help plan a smokefree night out to distract you.

## 6. Say thanks

Don't let acts of kindness go unnoticed. Tell your friends you appreciate them, whether you speak it, text it, or show it with your actions. Saying thanks doesn't take a lot of time, so do it in the moment before you forget.

**Tip:** Have a friend who gave up their last piece of gum to help you beat a cigarette craving? Buy some gum and give it to them with a note that says "Thanks for helping me stay quit!" Or tag them on Facebook so everyone knows how awesome they are.

### 7. Ditch the drama

Some people never have anything good to say and bring drama. Don't turn your life into a reality TV show. Steer clear of the things that add unneeded stress to your day and look for more positive things to do.

**Tip:** Pass on the trash talking and cigarette break after school. Stay above the fray by grabbing a friend and your sneakers and going for a walk instead.

### 8. Grow your social circle

Give your social circle a boost by connecting with other people who share your interests. Start by thinking about the things you like to do. Then look for ways to get more involved in them. Get talking with the people around you, and chances are, you'll find you have stuff in common.

**Tip:** Strike up a conversation with that kid who sits next to you in math class, join an after-school program, volunteer, or connect with the SfT Network.

### 9. Be approachable

How you present yourself to others is a big part of branching out and strengthening friendships. Make yourself approachable by making eye contact when talking with others. Smile. Sit and stand straight. Give compliments. People will be drawn to your confidence and positive attitude.

**Tip:** Say hi and smile to classmates when you pass them in the halls, compliment a random person on how great their shirt looks, or tell your friend you like their new haircut.

### 10. Set the stage

Don't wait around for others to come to you. Create opportunities to spend time with friends by suggesting things to do. Join in conversations and give your opinion (even if it's different from the rest). You don't have to be the center of attention to get noticed.

**Tip:** Approaching others might seem scary at first, so start small. Ask a classmate if you can sit with them at lunch or invite a friend over to play video games.

### 11. Listen

It's not always about you. Listening is a great way to strengthen and build friendships. Get people to open up by asking questions that can't be answered in just one word, like yes or no. Then be quiet and let them talk. Resist the urge to butt in with your own comments and stories.

**Tip:** Are your friend's eyes glazing over when you talk? Take a breath and give them a chance to say something. Ask what they think of a new song you heard or how they're feeling about semester exams.

### 12. Return the favor

Support is a two-way street. If you want others to be there for you, you have to be there for them, too. Check in with your friends and help them out when you can. Sometimes small favors mean the most.

**Tip:** Decorate a friend's locker to say good luck before a big game, send a tweet to recognize someone special, or make a friend smile by texting a random joke.

# Chapter 57

# How To Encourage Someone Who Is Trying To Quit Smoking

## How To Support Your Quitter

Someone who feels supported is more likely to quit smoking for good. That's why friends, family members, and significant others can play a big part in helping a person become smokefree.

Here are some tips that can help you support the person in your life who is quitting smoking. The more you know, the more you can help.

### It's Hard To Quit

Smoking cigarettes isn't a bad habit. It's a serious and complicated addiction. That makes quitting smoking one of the biggest challenges many smokers will ever face.

Deciding to quit doesn't mean thoughts of smoking go away at once. It takes time for cravings to fade, and it can take a person more than one try to successfully quit. Most people who quit don't do it on their own. They get a lot of help and support from friends, family, and significant others.

### Know Your Relationship Style

The way you deal with smoking can have an effect on a person who is trying to quit. It helps to become aware of your relationship style. Your style affects their smoking, their quitting, their health, and yours. Ask yourself these questions:

About This Chapter: This chapter includes text excerpted from "How To Support Your Quitter," Smokefree.gov, U.S. Department of Health and Human Services (HHS), July 20, 2016.

- Do you mind that they smoke around you?

- Do you argue about smoking?

- Do you avoid talking about smoking?

- Has a health problem changed the way you deal with smoking?

Understanding your relationship style can help you understand what both of you may have to change to better deal with their smoking and quitting. For example, you may need to:

- Recognize your friend or family member's small successes when quitting.

- Avoid criticizing them if they slip and have a cigarette.

- Decide it's time for you to quit smoking, too.

## Start The Conversation

It can be hard to get someone to talk about quitting smoking. To get a conversation started, look for an opening. Respond positively when someone says:

- I'm thinking about quitting smoking.

- My doctor told me that I should quit smoking.

- I'm pregnant. I should probably quit smoking.

- My wife is pregnant. I should probably quit smoking for her.

- My kids are asking me about my cigarettes. I should probably quit smoking for them.

Let them know you think it's great they're considering quitting and that you're ready to help. If you're an ex-smoker, you can draw from your own experience of quitting. Let them know how much better you feel now that you're smokefree. You might say:

- I'm so proud of you for trying to quit smoking. I'll help with whatever you need to make it happen.

- Quitting smoking will be hard, but I know you can do it. Have you set a quit date?

- You're not in this alone. Even if it gets tough, I'll be here for you.

- Quitting smoking is the best thing I ever did! Let me know if you need any tips.

## Create An Opening

If someone doesn't give you an opening, create one. Ask them whether they've thought about quitting. Or you could try a different approach. You might say:

- I heard on the news that taxes on cigarettes might go up soon. Sounds expensive. What do you think?

- I saw a commercial last night that showed an ex-smoker who lost teeth from gum disease caused by smoking. I didn't know that could happen. Did you?

## Ask Questions

Asking open-ended questions can help you understand what a smoker who is quitting is going through. You might ask:

- What made you want to start smoking?

- What things make you crave a cigarette?

- What made you decide to quit smoking?

- What things have been stressing you out lately?

- What could I do to help make quitting easier for you?

## Listen

Quitting smoking is about them—not you. Listen to what they have to say. If you ask a question, be quiet and give them time to answer. Resist the urge to insert your own comments.

## Don't Lecture

Lectures, nagging, and scolding won't help your friend or family member quit smoking. It might just put you on their bad side, and they may not come to you for help when they really need it.

Here are some things to avoid when you're trying to help someone quit smoking:

- Nagging them about why smoking is bad.

- Counting the number of cigarettes they smoked.

- Asking them if they smoked today.

- Arguing with them about being irritable when they're going through withdrawal.

- Giving them a hard time if they have a bigger appetite from withdrawal.

- Getting upset if they slip and smoke a cigarette.

## Offer Distractions

Lend support to your friend or family member by helping them plan smokefree activities. If you're still smoking, avoid smoking around them, especially if you call an activity "smokefree."

Here are a few activities you could suggest:

- Go to the movies (and let them choose the show).

- Take a walk.

- Plan a game night with a group of friends.

- Make dinner.

- Go out to eat at their favorite restaurant.

- Sign up for a class like photography, painting, or cooking.

- Go to a concert.

- Go to a basketball, baseball, or football game where smoking is not allowed.

Some triggers and cravings are unavoidable. Help your friend or family member prepare by thinking of ways to distract themselves until the craving passes. Most cravings only last a few minutes, so making a short phone call or finding a task to keep their hands busy might be enough.

Here are some ideas:

- Chew gum or slowly eat hard candy.

- Play a game on your cell phone. Which has games and challenges for distraction.

- Put a straw or toothpick in your mouth.

- Switch tasks for a change of scenery.

- Play with a rubber band.

- Munch on some carrot sticks, nuts, or celery.

- Squeeze a stress ball.

- Take deep breaths and try to relax.

- Drink lots of water.

Put together a smokefree quit kit with a few of these items for your friend or family member to help them be ready to deal with cravings in the moment.

## Be Patient And Positive

Supporting someone who is trying to quit smoking can be frustrating and exhausting. Focus on staying upbeat. Don't give up on them. Your support is important.

The withdrawal that can come from quitting smoking may make a person moody and irritable. Avoid:

- Taking their moods personally.

- Telling them it was easier to put up with their moods when they were smoking.

- Suggesting it would be easier for them to just go back to smoking.

The cravings a person might face can be hard to deal with. Don't let them lose confidence in quitting. Check in on them and let them know you support them. You might say:

- I can tell this is hard on you, but I'm proud of you for sticking with it. Let's do something fun to celebrate how far you've come!

- It sounds like you're having a rough day. How about I take care of dinner tonight/watch the kids/mow the lawn, so you can have some time for yourself? You deserve it.

## Don't Be Too Hard On Them If They Slip

Your friend or family member may slip at some point and smoke a cigarette. They'll probably feel guilty, so getting angry with them will not help. Instead, you could:

- Tell them you know they can still quit and remind them of all the progress they have made.

- Help them figure out what triggered the craving that led to the slip.

- Help them come up with a plan for dealing with the craving if it happens again.

- Ask if there is anything else you can do to help.

- Suggest they check out Smokefree's QuitGuide to keep track of when they slip and be aware of the things or places that are making quitting difficult.

Here are some ways you could respond to a slip:

- Slips happen. Don't beat yourself up over it! Like anything tough, you learn as you go. Use right now as a time to restart and get back on track.

- So you slipped. Quitting isn't easy and many people need several tries before they quit for good. You've got this, and I'm here for you.

- Let's talk about what's triggering you to smoke. That will help you stay on track this time. Just don't smoke that next cigarette!

## Celebrate Successes Big And Small

Recognize your friend or family member's smokefree successes and milestones. Staying smokefree for one day, one week, or one year are all reasons to celebrate. So are throwing out all of the ashtrays in the house, ditching any reminder of cigarettes, and passing on an after-dinner cigarette. Help your friend or family member celebrate by:

- Sending flowers or a card.

- Surprising them with tickets to a concert or show.

- Giving them a gift card to their favorite store.

- Making a home-cooked dinner.

A compliment can go a long way to recognize the positive changes they've made:

- The smokefree life works well for you—you look great!

- You make quitting smoking look easy. You should be proud of yourself. I am!

## Help Them De-Stress

Quitting smoking can create a lot of stress, which may cause someone to reach for a cigarette. If you notice they are stressed, help them break the cycle by finding healthier ways to de-stress. If you smoke, remember not to agree to have a cigarette together—that will set them back.

Consider suggesting one of these smokefree stress relievers:

- Close your eyes and take a few deep breaths.

- Play with a pet.

- Take a walk.

- Make a nice dinner.

- Read the Sunday comics.

- Try yoga or a spin class.

- Go to a comedy club or watch a funny TV show.

- Do a fun home project.

- Watch a sunset or sunrise.

- Do a crossword puzzle.

- Meet a friend at a cafe to chat.

- Take a nap.

- Take a bath or long shower.

## Be There For The Long Haul

The challenges of quitting smoking don't end when a person puts down their last cigarette. Cravings can pop up weeks, or even months, later. It's not uncommon for ex-smokers to start smoking again within the first three months of quitting.

Let your friend or family member know you're there for the long haul. Keep celebrating their smokefree anniversaries and offer distractions to help them deal with cravings. Your ongoing support could be all they need to make this quit attempt their last.

# Chapter 58

# Teen Smoking Prevention Campaigns

If you think smoking is part of a bygone, "Mad Men" era, think again. Young people, in particular, are still very much at risk. Every day in the United States more than 2,600 youth under age 18 smoke their first cigarette, and nearly 600 youth under age 18 become daily smokers.

As a regulator of tobacco products, U.S. Food and Drug Administration (FDA) also makes a strong commitment to educate the public (especially youth) about the harmful effects of using those products, says Kathleen Crosby, Director of the Office of Health Communication and Education (OHCE) at FDA's Center for Tobacco Products (CTP).

"The goal of our youth-oriented smoking prevention campaigns is to save kids' lives by helping them rethink their relationship with tobacco," she says. "For these kids, we're looking to disrupt their progression from thinking about smoking tobacco or starting to experiment with it, to becoming daily users." Through these campaigns, which have very distinct target audiences, FDA is looking to stop smoking behavior in its tracks.

## The Real Cost

The Real Cost, launched in 2014, is FDA's first national youth tobacco prevention campaign and its largest effort to date. The Real Cost aims to reach an estimated 10 million kids ages 12 to 17 who are open to smoking or already experimenting with cigarettes. In 2016, FDA plans to expand The Real Cost to include rural youth at risk of using smokeless tobacco.

---

About This Chapter: This chapter includes text excerpted from "FDA's Smoking Prevention Campaigns: Reaching Teens Where They 'Live,'" U.S. Food and Drug Administration (FDA), June 16, 2016.

## What Makes The Real Cost Unique?

"We're presenting new, research-based ideas that kids haven't heard before," Crosby says. To do so, The Real Cost uses provocative imagery and language kids can relate to, to dramatize the negative health consequences of smoking in a meaningful way and demonstrate that every cigarette comes with a "cost" that is more than just financial. For example, in one ad a teen is shown pulling out his own tooth to pay for a pack of cigarettes to highlight the potential consequence of tooth loss from smoking.

The Real Cost also makes active use of metaphors kids can relate to, such as equating tobacco addiction to having a bully in your life who is constantly telling you what to do and when to do it, something that FDA's research tells us is compelling to our independence-seeking target audience, Crosby says.

The Real Cost uses advertising on TV, radio and the Internet, as well as in print publications, movie theaters and outdoor locations like bus shelters.

The Real Cost is off to a great start. The campaign was awarded a gold Effie in the Disease Awareness and Education category at the 2015 North American Effie Awards as one of the most effective marketing efforts in the past year for its insightful communications strategy, outstanding creative, and success in market.

# Fresh Empire

Another targeted campaign effort—Fresh Empire—launched in fall 2015. Fresh Empire is the agency's first attempt at targeting underserved, multicultural populations, including African American, Hispanic, and Asian American/Pacific Islander youth.

"These are kids we know—from research on prevalence, demographics, and psychographics—identify strongly with the hip-hop culture. Smoking is commonly a part of that culture, and these teens are at high risk for it," Crosby says.

The campaign associates living tobacco-free with desirable hip-hop lifestyles. It uses a variety of interactive marketing tactics including the use of traditional paid media, engagement through multiple digital platforms, and outreach at the local level.

Both campaigns focus in on the dangers of addiction through loss of control, a persuasive message for youth who lead stressful lives, often magnified by low socioeconomic conditions and intensive peer pressure.

"Kids sometimes view tobacco as a way to cope with their problems and exert control over them," Cosby says. "We point out that by smoking, they actually cede control to tobacco, resulting in outcomes that negatively affect appearance, skin, teeth—we know from research are important to teens," Crosby says.

## Connecting Through Social Media

Both campaigns also make active use of social media on peer-to-peer platforms such as Facebook and Instagram. "We're reaching youth where they—sometimes quite literally—live and spend their time," Crosby says. "It brings credibility to our brand and enables us the opportunity to have one-on-one conversations." In fact, The Real Cost has resulted in more than two million conversations through social media platforms so far.

Moreover, social media also gives teens an opportunity to talk back and challenge the information presented. Crosby views this as a good thing.

"Many kids don't believe that they are (or will become) addicted—or that they'll suffer long-term health consequences like cancer," Crosby says. "These are new messages to youth, and they reach out for more information about it on social media, opening up a two-way dialogue that is more engaging and effective than, for example, a 30-second TV commercial might be."

## What's Next?

In May 2016, the agency released the "This Free Life" campaign, which is aimed at preventing and reducing tobacco use among lesbian, gay, bisexual and transgender (LGBT) young adults who are occasional smokers. And the FDA expanded the award-winning "The Real Cost" campaign to educate rural, white male teenagers about the negative health consequences associated with smokeless tobacco use.

In addition, FDA has set up a longitudinal evaluation study following thousands of kids over a 2-year period to determine if exposure to the campaign is contributing to a decrease in smoking among youth ages 12 to 17.

"Both the level of engagement we're seeing from teens on our social channels and our first two waves of evaluation data are promising," Crosby says. "Indications are that we're changing kids' attitudes and beliefs in the right direction."

# Part Six
## If You Need More Help Or Information

# Chapter 59

# Where To Get Help When You Decide To Quit Smoking

## Which Healthcare Professionals Can Help Me Quit Smoking?

Many healthcare professionals can be good sources of information about the health risks of smoking and the benefits of quitting. Talk to your doctor, dentist, pharmacist, or other healthcare provider about the proper use and potential side effects of nicotine replacement products and other medicines. They can also help you find local resources for assistance in quitting smoking.

## How Can I Find Out About National And Local Resources To Help Me Quit Smoking?

National Cancer Institute's (NCI) Smokefree.gov offers science-driven tools, information, and support that has helped smokers quit. You will find state and national resources, free materials, and quitting advice from NCI.

Smokefree.gov was established by the Tobacco Control Research Branch of NCI, a component of the National Institutes of Health (NIH), in collaboration with the Centers for Disease Control and Prevention (CDC) and other organizations.

Publications available from the Smokefree.gov Web site include the following:

- Clearing the Air: Quit Smoking Today for smokers interested in quitting.

About This Chapter: This chapter includes text excerpted from "Where To Get Help When You Decide To Quit Smoking," National Cancer Institute (NCI), October 28, 2010. Reviewed December 2016.

- Clear Horizons for smokers over age 50.

- Forever Free™ for smokers who have recently quit.

- Forever Free for Baby and Me™, in English and Spanish, for pregnant smokers who have recently quit.

- Clear Pathways: Winning the Fight Against Tobacco for African American smokers.

**NCI's Smoking Quitline** at **1–877–44U–QUIT (1–877–448–7848)** offers a wide range of services, including individualized counseling, printed information, referrals to other resources, and recorded messages. Smoking cessation counselors are available to answer smoking-related questions in English or Spanish, Monday through Friday, 8:00 a.m. to 8:00 p.m., Eastern time. Smoking cessation counselors are also available through LiveHelp, an online instant messaging service. LiveHelp is available Monday through Friday, 8:00 a.m. to 11:00 p.m., Eastern time.

Your state has a toll-free telephone quitline. Call **1–800–QUIT–NOW (1–800–784–8669)** to get one-on-one help with quitting, support and coping strategies, and referrals to resources and local cessation programs. The toll-free number routes callers to state-run quitlines, which provide free cessation assistance and resource information to all tobacco users in the United States. This initiative was created by the U.S. Department of Health and Human Services (HHS).

# Chapter 60

# The Health Effects Of Tobacco Use: A Directory Of Resources

## National and International Organizations

### Government Organizations

#### *Centers for Disease Control and Prevention (CDC)*

1600 Clifton Rd.
Atlanta, GA 30329-4027
Toll-Free: 800-CDC-INFO (800-232-4636)
TTY: 888-232-6348
Website: www.cdc.gov/tobacco

#### *National Cancer Institute (NCI)*

NCI Office of Communications and Education
Public Inquiries Office
9609 Medical Center Dr.
BG 9609 MSC 9760
Bethesda, MD 20892-9760
Toll-Free: 800-4-CANCER (800-422-6237)
TTY: 800-332-8615
Website: www.cancer.gov

Resources in this chapter were compiled from several sources deemed reliable, December 2016.

### National Heart, Lung, and Blood Institute (NHLBI)
NHLBI Health Information Center
P.O. Box 30105
Bethesda, MD 20824-0105
Phone: 301-592-8573
TTY: 240-629-3255
Website: www.nhlbi.nih.gov
E-mail: nhlbiinfo@nhlbi.nih.gov

### National Institute of Dental and Craniofacial Research (NIDCR)
Toll-Free: 866-232-4528
Website: www.nidcr.nih.gov
E-mail: nidcrinfo@mail.nih.gov

### National Institute of Mental Health (NIMH)
6001 Executive Blvd.
Rm. 6200, MSC 9663
Bethesda, MD 20892-9663
Toll-Free: 866-615-6464
Phone: 301-443-4536
Toll-Free TTY: 866-415-8051
TTY: 301-443-8431
Fax: 301-443-4279
Website: www.nimh.nih.gov
E-mail: nimhinfo@nih.gov

### National Institute on Drug Abuse (NIDA)
6001 Executive Blvd.
Rm. 5213, MSC 9561
Bethesda, MD 20892-9561
Phone: 301-443-1124
Website: www.nida.nih.gov

### Office of the Surgeon General
1101 Wootton Pkwy
Tower Bldg., Plaza Level 1, Rm. 100
Rockville, MD 20852
Phone: 202-205-0143
Fax: 240-453-6141
Website: www.surgeongeneral.gov
E-mail: ashmedia@hhs.gov

## Smokefree.gov

Tobacco Control Research Branch
9609 Medical Center Dr.
BG 9609 MSC 9760
Bethesda, MD 20892-9760
Phone: 301-496-8584
Fax: 301-496-8675
Website: smokefree.gov/privacy-policy
E-mail: NCISmokeFreeTeam@mail.nih.gov

## Substance Abuse and Mental Health Services Administration (SAMHSA)

5600 Fishers Ln.
P.O. Box 2345
Rockville, MD 20857
Toll-Free: 877-SAMHSA-7 (877-726-4727)
Toll-Free TDD: 800-487-4889
Fax: 240-221-4292
Website: www.samhsa.gov

## U.S. Department of Health and Human Services (HHS)

BeTobaccoFree.gov
200 Independence Ave., S.W.
Washington DC 20201
Website: betobaccofree.hhs.gov

## U.S. Environmental Protection Agency (EPA)

1200 Pennsylvania Ave., N.W.
Washington, DC 20460
Website: www.epa.gov

## U.S. Food and Drug Administration (FDA)

Center for Tobacco Products
10903 New Hampshire Ave.
Bldg. 71, Rm. G335
Silver Spring, MD 20993-0002
Toll-Free: 877-CTP-1373 (877-287-1373)
Phone: 301-796-9270
Website: www.fda.gov
E-mail: AskCTP@fda.hhs.gov

## Private Organizations

### *Action on Smoking and Health (ASH)*

1250 Connecticut Ave., N.W.
Washington, DC 20036
Phone: 202-659-4310
Website: ash.org
E-mail: info@ash.org

### *American Academy of Family Physicians (AAFP)*

11400 Tomahawk Creek Pkwy
Leawood, KS 66211-2680
Toll-Free: 800-274-2237
Phone: 913-906-6000
Fax: 913-906-6075
Website: www.aafp.org
E-mail: aafp@aafp.org

### *American Cancer Society (ACS)*

250 Williams St., N.W.
Atlanta, GA 30303
Toll-Free: 800-ACS-2345 (800-227-2345)
Website: www.cancer.org

### *American College of Chest Physicians*

CHEST Global Headquarters
2595 Patriot Blvd.
Glenview, IL 60026
Toll-Free: 800-343-2227
Phone: 224-521-9800
Fax: 224-521-9801
Website: www.chestnet.org

### *American Council on Science and Health (ACSH)*

110 E. 42nd St.
Ste. 1300
New York, NY 10017
Phone: 212-362-7044
Website: www.acsh.org
E-mail: acsh@acsh.org

## American Dental Hygienists' Association (ADHA)

444 N. Michigan Ave.
Ste. 3400
Chicago, IL 60611
Phone: 312-440-8900
Website: www.adha.org

## American Heart Association (AHA)

National Center
7272 Greenville Ave.
Dallas, TX 75231
Toll-Free: 800-AHA-USA1 (800-242-8721)
Website: www.heart.org
E-mail: Review.personal.info@heart.org

## American Lung Association (ALA)

National Office
55 W. Wacker Dr.
Ste. 1150
Chicago, IL 60601
Toll-Free: 800-LUNG-USA (800-548-8252)
Website: www.lung.org
E-mail: info@lung.org

## American Public Health Association (APHA)

800 I St., N.W.
Washington, DC 20001
Phone: 202-777-APHA (202-777-2742)
TTY: 202-777-2500
Fax: 202-777-2534
Website: www.apha.org

## Americans for Nonsmokers' Rights (ANR)

2530 San Pablo Ave.
Ste. J
Berkeley, CA 94702
Phone: 510-841-3032
Fax: 510-841-3071
Website: www.no-smoke.org

### The BADvertising Institute

Phone: 207-420-1434
Website: www.badvertising.org
E-mail: bv@badvertising.org

### Bureau of Tobacco Free Florida (BTFF)

4052 Bald Cypress Way
Bin C-23
Tallahassee, FL 32399-1743
Phone: 850-245-4144
Website: www.tobaccofreeflorida.com
E-mail: contact@tobaccofreeflorida.com

### Campaign for Tobacco-Free Kids

1400 Eye St., N.W.
Ste. 1200
Washington, DC 20005
Phone: 202-296-5469
Fax: 202-296-5427
Website: www.tobaccofreekids.org

### Canadian Council for Tobacco Control (CCTC)

192 Bank St.
Ottawa, ON K2P 1W8
Canada
Toll-Free: 800-267-5234
Phone: 613-567-3050
Website: www.cctc.ca
E-mail: info-services@cctc.ca

### Canadian Lung Association (CLA)

1750 Courtwood Crescent
Ste. 300
Ottawa, ON K2C 2B5
Canada
Toll-Free: 888-566-LUNG (888-566-5864)
Phone: 613-569-6411
Website: www.lung.ca
E-mail: info@lung.ca

### The Center for Social Gerontology (TCSG)

2307 Shelby Ave.
Ann Arbor, MI 48103
Phone: 734-665-1126
Fax: 734-665-2071
Website: www.tcsg.org
E-mail: tcsg@tcsg.org

### The Foundation for a Smokefree America

8117 W. Manchester Ave.
Ste. 500
Playa del Rey, CA 90293-8745
Phone: 310-577-9828
Fax: 310-388-1350
Website: www.anti-smoking.org
E-mail: contact@anti-smoking.org

### Group Against Smog and Pollution (GASP)

1133 S. Braddock Ave.
Ste. 1A
Edgewood, PA 15218
phone: 412-924-0604
Website: www.gasp-pgh.org
E-mail: info@gasp-pgh.org

### National Families in Action (NFIA)

P.O. Box 133136
Atlanta, GA 30333-3136
Phone: 404-248-9676
Website: www.nationalfamilies.org
E-mail: nfia@nationalfamilies.org

### The Ohio State University Wexner Medical Center (OSUMC)

410 W. 10th Ave.
Columbus, OH 43210
Phone: 614-293-8000
Website: wexnermedical.osu.edu
E-mail: OSUCareConnection@osumc.edu

## Partnership For A Tobacco-Free Maine (PTM)

Maine Department of Health and Human Services
11 State House Stn
Key Bank Plaza, 4th Fl.
Augusta, ME 04330-0011
Toll-Free: 800-207-1230
Phone: 207-287-4627
Fax: 207-287-4636
Website: www.tobaccofreemaine.org
E-mail: ptm.dhhs@maine.gov

## Partnership for Drug-Free Kids

352 Park Ave., S.
9th Fl.
New York, NY 10010
Toll-Free: 855-DRUGFREE (855-378-4373)
Phone: 212-922-1560
Fax: 212-922-1570
Website: www.drugfree.org

## Public Health Law Center

Mitchell Hamline School of Law
875 Summit Ave.
St. Paul, MN 55105
Phone: 651-290-7506
Fax: 651-290-7515
Website: publichealthlawcenter.org
E-mail: publichealthlaw@mitchellhamline.edu

## Robert Wood Johnson Foundation (RWJF)

College Rd. E. and Rt. 1
P.O. Box 2316
Princeton, NJ 08543-2316
Toll-Free: 877-843-RWJF (877-843-7953)
Website: www.rwjf.org

### Society for Research on Nicotine and Tobacco (SRNT)
2424 American Ln.
Madison, WI 53704
Phone: 608-443-2462
Fax: 608-443-2474
Website: www.srnt.org
E-mail: info@srnt.org

### Tobacco Free Allegheny
1501 Reedsdale St.
The Cardello Bldg., Ste. 2006
Pittsburgh, PA 15233
Phone: 412-322-TFA1 (412-322-8321)
Fax: 412-322-TFA3 (412-322-8323)
Website: www.tobaccofreeallegheny.org

### TobaccoFreeCA
CA Department of Public Health
P.O. Box 997377
Sacramento, CA 95899-737
Website: tobaccofreeca.com

### Tobacco Technical Assistance Consortium (TTAC)
Emory University
1599 Clifton Rd.
6th Fl. MS: 1599-001-1BW
Atlanta, GA 30322
Phone: 404-712-8474
Fax: 404-712-8766
Website: www.ttac.org
E-mail: ttac@sph.emory.edu

### University of Wisconsin Center for Tobacco Research and Intervention (UW-CTRI)
1930 Monroe St.
Ste. 200
Madison, WI 53711
Phone: 608-262-8673
Website: www.ctri.wisc.edu
E-mail: infoctri@ctri.wisc.edu

### U.S. Bureau of Alcohol, Tobacco, Firearms, and Explosives (ATF)

Office of Public and Governmental Affairs
99 New York Ave., N.E.
Washington, DC 20226
Toll Free: 800-800-3855
Phone: 202-648-7777
Website: www.atf.gov
E-mail: ATFTips@atf.gov

### Virginia Smoke Free Association (VSFA)

10104 Chester Rd.
Chester, VA 23831
Phone: 804-318-9183
Website: virginiasmokefree.org
E-mail: info@virginiasmokefree.org

# Chapter 61
# Smoking Cessation Resources

## Cessation Help By Phone

**American Cancer Society (ACS)**
Toll-Free: 800-ACS-2345 (800-227-2345)

**American Heart Association (AHA)**
Toll-Free: 800-AHA-USA-1 (800-242-8721)

**American Lung Association (ALA)**
Toll-Free: 800-LUNG-USA (800-586-4871)

**American Stroke Association (ASA)**
Toll-Free: 888-4-STROKE (888-478-7653)

**Arizona Smokers' Helpline (ASHLine)**
Toll-Free: 800-556-6222

**Illinois Tobacco Quitline (ITQ)**
Toll-Free: 866-QUIT-YES (866-784-8937)

**National Network of Tobacco Cessation Quitlines (NNTCQ)**
Toll-Free: 800-QUITNOW (800-784-8669)

**New York State Smokers' Quitline**
Toll-Free: 866-NY-QUITS (866-697-8487)

---

Resources in this chapter were compiled from several sources deemed reliable, December 2016.

**Nicotine Anonymous (NicA)**
Toll-Free: 877-TRY-NICA (877-879-6422)

**Office on Smoking & Health (OSH)**
Toll-Free: 800-CDC-INFO (800-232-4636)

**Smokers Helpline**
Toll-Free: 877-513-5333

**Smoking Quitline**
Toll-Free: 877-44U-QUIT (877-448-7848)

**TRICARE®'s Smoking QuitLine**
Toll-Free: North Region: 866-459-8766 | South Region: 877-414-9949 | West Region: 888–713–4597

**QUITPLAN Helpline**
888-354-PLAN (888-354-7526)

**Quitting Smoking**
Toll-Free: 877-455-2233

# Online Resources

**Center for Tobacco Cessation (CTC)**
Website: www.ctcinfo.org

**Coalition for Tobacco-Free Arizona (CTFA)**
Website: www.tobaccofreeaz.org

**Committed Quitters**
Website: www.quit.com

**Help for Smokers and Other Tobacco Users**
Website: www.ahrq.gov/professionals/clinicians-providers/guidelines-recommendations/tobacco/clinicians/tearsheets/helpsmokers.html

**Helping Young Smokers Quit**
Website: www.helpingyoungsmokersquit.org

**Kick Butts Day (KBD)**
Website: www.kickbuttsday.org

### My Last Dip
Website: www.mylastdip.com

### National Lung Health Education Program (NLHEP)
Website: www.nlhep.org

### Nicotine Anonymous (NicA)
Website: www.nicotine-anonymous.org

### The Partnership for a Drug-Free Kids
Website: www.drugfree.org

### Quit Tobacco. Make Everyone Proud
Website: www.ucanquit2.org

### Quit Plan
Website: www.quitplan.com

### QuitNet
Website: www.quitnet.com

### Smokefree Families
Website: tobacco-cessation.org/sf

### Smokefree
Website: www.smokefree.gov

### Smokefree Teen
Website: Teen.Smokefree.gov

### Smokefree Women
Website: women.smokefree.gov

### University of Rochester
Website: www.rochester.edu

### Why Quit
Website: www.whyquit.com

### Youth Quit 4 Life
Website: www.quit4life.com

### Youth Tobacco Cessation Collaborative (YTCC)
Website: www.youthtobaccocessation.org

## Smokefree Mobile Apps

### LIVESTRONG My Quit Coach
Website: www.livestrong.com/mobile-apps

### Quit It Lite
Website: www.digitalsirup.com/app/quitit/?lang=en

### Quit Smoking
Website: quit.azati.com

### Quit Smoking: Cessation Nation
Website: wearecessationnation.com

### QuitNow
Website: quitnowapp.com/en

### Smoke Free App
Website: smokefreeapp.com

# Index

# Index

Page numbers that appear in *Italics* refer to tables or illustrations. Page numbers that have a small 'n' after the page number refer to citation information shown as Notes. Page numbers that appear in **Bold** refer to information contained in boxes within the chapters.